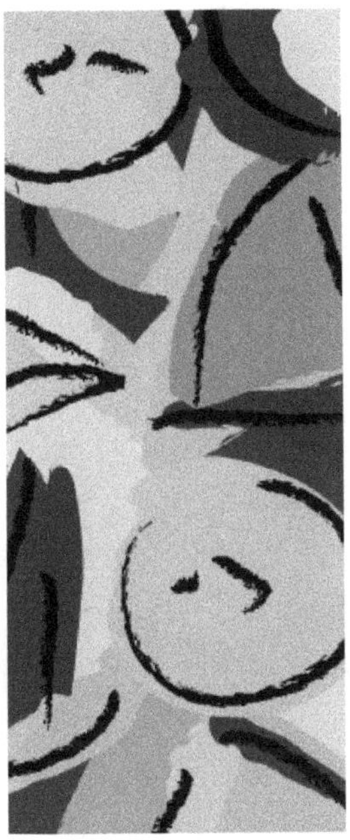

MacArthur Inventarios del Desarrollo de Habilidades Comunicativas

User's Guide and Technical Manual

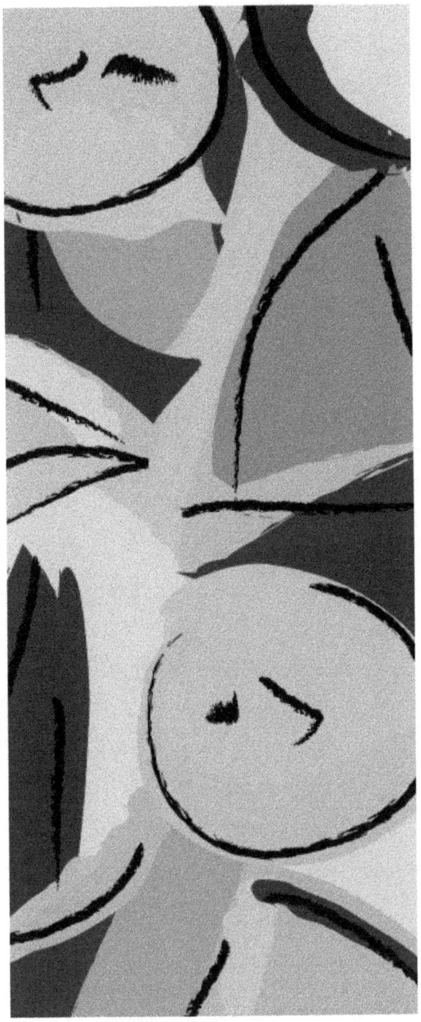

MacArthur Inventarios del Desarrollo de Habilidades Comunicativas

User's Guide and Technical Manual

MacArthur INVENTARIOS

by

Donna Jackson-Maldonado, Ph.D.

Donna J. Thal, Ph.D.

Virginia A. Marchman, Ph.D.

Larry Fenson, Ph.D.

Tyler Newton, M.A.

Barbara Conboy, Ph.D.

PAUL H. BROOKES PUBLISHING CO.®

Baltimore • London • Sydney

Paul H. Brookes Publishing Co.
Post Office Box 10624
Baltimore, Maryland 21285-0624

www.brookespublishing.com

Typeset by A.W. Bennett, Inc., Hartland, Vermont.

To learn more about the *MacArthur Inventarios,*
go to www.brookespublishing.com.

This manual accompanies the *MacArthur Inventarios del Desarrollo de Habilidades Comunicativas,* which may be purchased in packages of 25. To order, contact Paul H. Brookes Publishing Co. (1-800-638-3775; 410-337-9580; custserv@brookespublishing.com).

Library of Congress Cataloging-in-Publication Data

MacArthur Inventarios del Desarrollo de Habilidades Comunicativas:
user's guide and technical manual / by Donna Jackson-Maldonado . . .
[et al.].
p. cm.
Includes bibliographical references and index.
ISBN 1-55766-617-2
1. Language acquisition—Testing. 2. Language acquisition—Parent
participation. 3. MacArthur Communicative Development
Inventories. I. Jackson-Maldonado, Donna.
P118.75.M33 2003
418′.0076—dc21 2003041789

British Library Cataloguing in Publication data are available from the British Library.

CONTENTS

LIST OF TABLES AND FIGURES

THE CDI ADVISORY BOARD

***Chair,* Larry Fenson, Ph.D.**
Department of Psychology
San Diego State University
lfenson@sunstroke.sdsu.edu

Elizabeth Bates, Ph.D.
Department of Cognitive Science
University of California, San Diego
bates@crl.ucsd.edu

Philip S. Dale, Ph.D.
Department of Communication Science and Disorders
University of Missouri at Columbia
dalep@health.missouri.edu

Donna Jackson-Maldonado, Ph.D.
Department of Languages and Literature (Facultad de Lenguas y Letras)
Universidad Autónoma de Querétaro
Mexico
djackson@sunserver.dsi.uaq.mx

Virginia A. Marchman, Ph.D.
School of Behavioral and Brain Sciences
The University of Texas at Dallas
vamarch@utdallas.edu

J. Steven Reznick, Ph.D.
Department of Psychology
University of North Carolina at Chapel Hill
reznick@unc.edu

Donna J. Thal, Ph.D.
School of Speech, Language, and Hearing Sciences
San Diego State University
dthal@mail.sdsu.edu

ABOUT THE AUTHORS

Donna Jackson-Maldonado, Ph.D., Professor, Department of Languages and Literature (Facultad de Lenguas y Letras), Universidad Autónoma de Querétaro, Qa de Cedros 676, 76100 Mexico

Dr. Jackson-Maldonado was born in the United States but was brought up in Mexico. She has lived in a bilingual-bicultural environment all of her life. Her initial professional experience was as a speech-language pathologist working with children with language disorders and learning disabilities and deaf children. She also has worked for the Mexican government's special education and communication disorders programs, doing in-service training, writing books and manuals, and developing language assessment instruments.

Dr. Jackson-Maldonado received her doctorate in linguistics from El Colegio de México in Mexico City. Her research has been in Spanish and bilingual language development in infants and toddlers. Part of this work was the development of the MacArthur Inventarios del Desarrollo de Habilidades Comunicativas and, with Donna J. Thal, a language and gesture battery for Spanish speakers.

Dr. Jackson-Maldonado is currently a full-time professor and researcher at the Universidad Autónoma de Querétaro in Mexico. She directs a project on late-talking Spanish-speaking toddlers.

Donna J. Thal, Ph.D., Professor, School of Speech, Language, and Hearing Sciences, San Diego State University (SDSU), and Research Psychologist, Center for Research in Language, University of California, San Diego (UCSD), 6330 Alvarado Court, Suite 231, San Diego, California 92120-1850

Dr. Thal holds a master of science degree in speech pathology and audiology from Brooklyn College and a doctorate in speech and hearing sciences from the Graduate School and University Center of the City University of New York (CUNY). She has been a postdoctoral fellow at the Center for Research in Language at UCSD, an assistant professor at Hofstra University, and an assistant professor at Queens College of CUNY. Dr. Thal is a developmental psycholinguist and a certified and licensed speech-language pathologist who has conducted research in a number of areas, including normal and disordered development of language and cognition, children with focal brain injury, and children with delayed onset of language. She has also carried out studies of language development in Spanish-speaking infants and toddlers. Her most recent work focuses on early identification of risk for clinically significant language impairment and is funded by a grant from the National Institute of Deafness and Other Communicative Disorders (NIDCD), within the National Institutes of Health.

Dr. Thal is an editorial consultant for language for the *Journal of Speech, Language, and Hearing Research* and the *American Journal of Speech-Language Pathology.* She was the California State nominee for the American Speech-Language-Hearing Foundation Outstanding Clinical Achievement Award in 1996, received the Monty Distinguished Faculty Award from SDSU 1998 and the Albert W. Johnson Research Lecturer Award from SDSU in 1999, and was the Wang Family Excellence Award nominee from SDSU in 2000. She served a 4-year term on the Communicative Disorders Review Committee for the NIDCD from 1998 to 2002. Dr. Thal is a co-author of the MacArthur Communicative Development Inventories.

Virginia A. Marchman, Ph.D., Associate Professor, School of Behavioral and Brain Sciences, Post Office Box 830688 GR 41, The University of Texas at Dallas, Richardson, Texas 75083-0688

Dr. Marchman holds a master of arts degree and a doctorate in developmental psychology from the University of California, Berkeley. She has been an assistant professor at the University of Wisconsin, Madison, and a postdoctoral fellow at the Center for Research in Language at the University of California, San Diego. She has conducted research in several areas of language and cognitive development, language disorders, and early childhood development. Her most recent work focuses on the identification of precursors of language delay and individual differences in lexical and morphological development in monolingual English and bilingual (Spanish and English) speakers. She is on the editorial board of the *Journal of Speech, Language, and Hearing Research* and was named Distinguished Scholar at the Callier Center for Communication Disorders. Dr. Marchman has worked on the MacArthur Communicative Development Inventories and the MacArthur Inventarios del Desarrollo de Habilidades Comunicativas for the last 15 years. She is author of the CDI Scoring Program (http://www.sci.sdsu.edu/cdi/scoringdb_p.htm).

Larry Fenson, Ph.D., Professor of Psychology, San Diego State University, 6505 Alvarado, Suite 101, San Diego, California 92120-5010

Dr. Fenson has published research on infant attentiveness, early symbolic development, categorization, children's drawing skills, play, and early language development. He received his doctorate in child psychology from the University of Iowa. He served as Assistant Professor at the University of Denver and was a National Institute of Child Health and Human Development postdoctoral fellow with Jerome Kagan at Harvard University. Dr. Fenson is Chair of The CDI Advisory Board.

Tyler Newton, M.A., Teacher, 39639 Old Highway 80, Clover Flat Elementary School, Boulevard, California 91905-9733

Tyler Newton received bachelor of arts and master of arts degrees in psychology from San Diego State University. She obtained the California Multiple Subject Teaching Credential from San Diego State University in 2000 and currently teaches second and third grades at Clover Flat Elementary School in Boulevard, California. Her master's thesis involved work on the norming study for the MacArthur Inventarios del Desarrollo de Habilidades Comunicativas.

Barbara Conboy, Ph.D., Center for Mind, Brain & Learning, University of Washington, Box 357988, Seattle, Washington 98195-7988

Dr. Conboy is currently a postdoctoral research associate at the Center for Mind, Brain & Learning at the University of Washington. She earned a doctorate in language and communicative disorders at the University of California, San Diego/San Diego State University; a master of arts degree in speech-language-hearing at Temple University; and a bachelor of arts in Latin American studies at Smith College. She is certified by the American Speech-Language-Hearing Association as a speech-language pathologist and has worked extensively with bilingual children with language-learning disorders. Her research interests include early bilingualism, experiential factors in language acquisition and brain development, and the early identification and treatment of language impairment in bilingual children.

ACKNOWLEDGMENTS

We wish to thank the students and research assistants at the three study sites for various contributions to collecting the forms, scanning and coding the data, entering data, maintaining records, assisting with data analysis, and preparing the manuscript of the user's guide and technical manual. *In San Diego:* Dora Acosta, Luz Angel, Teresa Colín, and Marjorie Palacios. *In Mexico:* Julia Barragán Trejo, Rosa Patricia Bárcenas Acosta, Gabriela Carrillo Aranguren, Jesús Alfonso Chávez Velarde, Claudia Díaz Molina, Lourdes Fernández Solis, Araceli García Olvera, Rocío Jaime Domínguez, Maria Carmen López Gómez, Elizabeth Rivera, Martha Beatriz Soto Martínez, and Yesenia Trejo Trejo. *In Dallas:* Lori Carrizal, Elda Jimenez, Carmen Martínez-Sussmann, and Laura Smithson. Thanks also to Steven Pethick for technical support.

We thank our colleagues for their advice and assistance: Philip S. Dale, Vera Gutiérrez-Clellen, Ricardo Maldonado, and especially Elizabeth Bates, who had the ideas that gave birth to the original MacArthur Communicative Development Inventories and who nurtured the development of the Inventarios from infancy through maturity.

We would like to express our appreciation to all of the parents who so generously gave their time. We would also like to thank the staffs of the Day Care Centers of the National Institute of Social Security (IMSS), Giocare, Buckingham, Infantes y Crayolas, Brincos, and Traviesos y Traviesas child care centers in Querétaro, Mexico, and those of the OIRA Center of the University of the Americas and Siglo XXI in Mexico City. We also appreciate the help of the pediatricians in Querétaro, Mexico, who referred children to our study. In the United States, we thank Susan Nevitt of the Logan Heights Family Health Center in San Diego, California, and the staff of the Women, Infants, and Children (WIC) program administered by the County of San Diego. We are also grateful to the staff at Paul H. Brookes Publishing Co. for their careful editing and many helpful suggestions with regard to the form of the manual.

The project on which this manual is based was partially funded by the MacArthur Foundation Research Network on Childhood Transitions, grants from the Consejo Nacional de Ciencia y Tecnología and UC-MEXUS, and funds from the Universidad Autónoma de Querétaro in Mexico to support research assistants. We thank all of these institutions for their generosity in helping us to develop the Inventarios.

To Liz Bates
for her creativity, enthusiasm, and support

1

INTRODUCTION

OVERVIEW

Since the early 1990s, parent[1] report has found widespread use as a method for measuring language development in clinical practice and in research. Commonly used laboratory and clinical measures such as structured testing and language sampling require a substantial commitment of trained personnel and time that is often not feasible in research studies involving large numbers of children or in clinical evaluations of individual children. Parent report instruments provide an alternative to such measures by utilizing the knowledge that most parents and caregivers have about their young children's language development. When tapped appropriately, parents' knowledge can assist clinicians and researchers in determining children's levels of language development and thus can lead to a more ecologically valid assessment (Crais, 1995). Such measures are also responsive to Part C of the Individuals with Disabilities Education Act (IDEA) Amendments of 1997 (PL 105-17), which requires parent input in evaluation procedures for young children.

The publication of the MacArthur Communicative Development Inventories (CDIs; Fenson et al., 1992/1993; Fenson, Pethick, et al., 2000) has allowed valid and efficient measurement of specific vocabulary and morphosyntactic forms by English-speaking children ages 8–30 months. The CDIs have been used in a wide array of settings and disciplines and have been adapted and normed for use with many different language groups (see the page about adaptations that appears on the CDI web site, http://www.sci.sdsu.edu/cdi/foreign.html, for a complete list). These adaptations are not mere translations to other languages but rather are versions that take linguistic and cultural differences into account. Many of the adaptations have been normed on samples of children from the particular cultural and linguistic group in question. Norming and validation have also been completed for a CDI-III in English, a short form of the CDI to be used with children 30–38 months of age (Dale, Reznick, & Thal, 1998).

[1]In this manual, the term *parents* refers to a child's parents or primary caregivers.

The use of parent report among practitioners and researchers has increased considerably since the early 1990s. Practitioners have found that parent report measures are useful in screening and developing a prognosis for children with language delays (Crais, 1995; Rescorla, 1991; Yoder, Warren, & McCathren, 1998). Still, caution has been recommended regarding use of parent report as the sole measure for identifying children with language disorders. There is general consensus that multiple measures are needed for this purpose. Researchers have also found parent report to be useful for establishing levels of language proficiency for contrast to other cognitive skills within groups or for comparisons across groups of children. Parent report has now been used extensively in research with a wide variety of children, including children with language delay, children with Down and Williams syndromes, bilingual children, children in daytime care, children from different socioeconomic groups, and infants who were born preterm or with focal lesions. (See the section in Chapter 2 called "Using the Norms with Children from Families of Low Socioeconomic Status" and the section in Chapter 3 called "Evaluation of Older Children with Language Delay.")

The instruments described in this manual, the MacArthur Inventarios del Desarrollo de Habilidades Comunicativas, are Spanish adaptations of the English (Fenson et al., 1992/1993) and Italian (Caselli & Casadio, 1995) CDIs. Both of those CDIs were based on the Early Language Inventory (Bates et al., 1985). These Spanish adaptations have been developed specifically for Spanish-speaking children, using normative data collected over 9 years in Mexico (see the section in Chapter 4 called "Phases of Development of the Inventarios"). *Primeras Palabras y Gestos* (First Words and Gestures; hereafter referred to as Inventario I) is designed for 8- to 18-month-olds and generates scores for comprehension of words and phrases, vocabulary production, and use of gestures. *Palabras y Enunciados* (Words and Sentences; hereafter referred to as Inventario II) is designed for 16- to 30-month-olds and yields scores for vocabulary production and a number of aspects of grammatical development, including sentence complexity, verb conjugations, and mean length (in words) of three of the child's longest utterances. The norms provided in Chapter 5 permit a child's scores on each of the major components of the inventories to be converted to percentile values, reflecting the child's relative rank to other children of the same age and sex.

Organization of This Manual

This manual has been written in the same format as the English CDI *User's Guide and Technical Manual* (Fenson et al., 1992/1993), for the convenience of users who are already familiar with the English CDIs. The general structure of the instruments, as well as many of the administration and scoring techniques, are the same as presented in the English CDI manual. Because of important sociolinguistic and sociocultural differences, however, the Inventarios themselves, their administration, and their scoring differ from the English CDIs in several important respects. It is therefore imperative that users of the Inventarios become familiar with this *User's Guide and Technical Manual,* regardless of their familiarity or degree of previous experience with the English CDIs and their accompanying manual (Fenson et al., 1992/1993).

The main body of this manual is divided into five chapters. In Chapter 1, methods of assessing early language development are reviewed, the role and value of parent report are considered, and the instruments themselves are described. (In this detailed description of the Inventarios and in the rest of this manual, the titles of the corresponding categories on the English CDIs are provided in square brackets, such as *Lista de Vocabulario* [Vocabulary Checklist]. Glosses are also provided in square brackets for parts of the Inventarios that have no analogous section on the English CDIs; these glosses are preceded by an asterisk.) In Chapter 2, directions for administering, scoring, and interpreting the inventories are provided. In Chapter 3, possible applications of the inventories for clinical and research purposes are outlined. In Chapter 4, background information on the development of the Spanish instruments is furnished, details of the developmental trends for the norming sample are presented, the correlations among the various components of each inventory are described, and measures of the reliability and validity of the instruments are reported. Finally, Chapter 5 presents percentile tables and figures for major variables separately for boys and girls and for both sexes combined.

This manual's appendices provide accompanying forms for gathering demographic information (Appendix A, Basic Information Form and *Forma de Información Básica*) and supplemental handouts with instructions to parents (Appendix B, General Instructions and *Instrucciones Generales*). Appendix C (Further Instructions and Examples) summarizes instructions to parents regarding acceptable variants of items on the *Lista de Vocabulario* [Vocabulary Checklist] of each Inventario. Appendices D and E (Scoring Examples for Inventario I, and Scoring Examples for Inventario II and Scoring Guidelines for *M3L-Palabras* [M3L-*Words], respectively) provide examples for scoring several key sections of the Inventarios, including specific guidelines for the computation of the mean length in words of the three longest utterances, *M3L-Palabras* [M3L-*Words]. A description of items in the *Complejidad de Frases* [Complexity] section is provided in Appendix F. Finally, Appendix G (Child Report Forms and *Informes del Niño/a*) provides templates for reporting scores in English and Spanish, respectively.

METHODS OF ASSESSING EARLY LANGUAGE SKILLS IN SPANISH-SPEAKING CHILDREN

The language assessment techniques used in research and clinical assessment of Spanish-speaking infants and toddlers have paralleled those used with children of other language backgrounds. These techniques fall into three categories: structured tests, language samples, and parent report. Each of these is discussed next.

Structured Tests

In structured tests, responses are elicited from the child in a relatively formal manner in order to assess the child's knowledge of vocabulary and grammar. The limitations of structured tests often outweigh their benefits when used with infants and toddlers. Tests require time, trained personnel, and the cooperation of the young child. As Fenson and colleagues (1992/1993) have commented, the usefulness of structured tests is also limited by their expense, the modest validity that most of these instruments show when used with children younger than 2½–3 years of age, and the inherent problems that arise when the instruments are used on linguistically and culturally diverse populations (Crais, 1995; Gutierrez-Clellen, 1996; Kayser, 1995; Lahey, 1988; Langdon, 1992a, 1992b; Mattes & Omark, 1991). Furthermore, very few tests have been developed specifically for Spanish-speaking infants or toddlers. Most of those that exist are direct translations of English tests, such as the Sequenced Inventory of Communicative Development–Spanish Translation (Hedrick, Prather, & Tobin, 1984) and the Expressive One-Word Picture Vocabulary Test–Revised, Spanish Version (Gardner, 1990). The Preschool Language Scale–3, Spanish Edition (PLS-3 Spanish Edition; Zimmerman, Steiner, & Pond, 1993b) is also a direct translation of the English form (Zimmerman, Steiner, & Pond, 1993a) but now has Spanish norms. Others, such as the Test de Vocabulario en Imágenes Peabody, Adaptación Hispanoamericana (Dunn, Lugo, Padilla, & Dunn, 1986), are not direct translations but rather are adaptations that are modeled after English tests and normed on Spanish-speaking populations in the United States and elsewhere. Unfortunately, these have limited construct validity because their content and structure do not necessarily reflect the order of acquisition of lexical and morphosyntactic items in Spanish-speaking populations (see Gutierrez-Clellen, 1996; Jackson-Maldonado, 1988, 1999; and Langdon, 1992b, for discussions of this issue). Of the few standardized language tests that have been developed and normed with Mexican children, only one, the Sistema de Evaluación Sobre la Adquisición de la Lengua Española (Merino, Figueroa, Gómez Palacio, Rangel Hinojosa, & Jackson-Maldonado, 1987), has been normed on a group of children between the ages of 2 and 11 years (thus including toddlers).

Language Samples

Language sampling is a second popular technique that is used by researchers and clinicians who work with children from a variety of language communities and cultures. A typical language sample is gathered in a naturalistic play context with the child and a parent, an experimenter, or a clinician. Parents are asked to play with their child as they would at home. Experimenters and clinicians are trained to follow the child's lead, to make conversational responses to the child's utterances, and to ask open-ended questions. Transcription and analysis of naturalistic language samples require highly trained personnel and a substantial amount of time. As a result, most studies incorporating language samples use small numbers of children. Special care needs to be taken when generalizing results from case studies or when data are obtained from a small sample. Another complication with language sampling is that the behavior observed during interactions is highly variable across contexts and interlocutors. In all interactions between a child and another person, it is the dyad that is assessed. Clearly, parent–child interactions will differ from exchanges between a child and a specifically trained clinician or researcher. Interactions will also differ across parents and across clinicians/researchers, regardless of the level of training. In addition, context has a strong effect, especially with young children. The characteristics of the observations of a child with a parent at home are likely to differ from those carried out in a laboratory or clinic.

Although a language sample may yield a broader reflection of a child's vocabulary and grammar than a structured test might reveal, the method still assesses a restricted range of the child's abilities. Researchers and clinicians are often most interested in emerging skills. It is precisely those skills that are unlikely to be observed in a spontaneous play interaction in which the interlocutor will tend to follow the child's lead and purposely refrain from asking pointed or difficult questions.

An additional complication of using language samples with Spanish-speaking children reflects the fact that this technique was developed in the United States with middle-income children who are likely to have had extensive experience with these types of interactions (e.g., Bloom & Lahey, 1978; Lund & Duchan, 1988; Miller, 1981; van Kleeck & Richardson, 1990). Free play with adults, however, may be an unfamiliar situation for children from cultural groups in which such interactions may be a less common practice in the home (Delgado-Gaitán & Trueba, 1991; Farver, 1993; Heath, 1983; Roopnarine, Johnson, & Hooper, 1994; see also Langdon, 1992a, 1992b, for a discussion of this issue). Furthermore, investigators have demonstrated that the types of language functions that are observed during adult–child interactions vary across situations and sociocultural groups (e.g., Bavin, 1992; Blount, 1978; Bornstein & Haynes, 1998; Bornstein, Haynes, & Paynter, 1998; Bornstein, Tamis-LeMonda, & Haynes, 1999; Demuth, 1992; Farver, 1993; Heath, 1983, 1986; Iglesias, 1985; Ochs, 1982; Schieffelin & Eisenberg, 1984; Schieffelin & Ochs, 1986; Zukow, 1984; Zukow-Goldring, 2001). Language samples are highly sensitive to the fact that children from different cultures are likely to vary in the types of language or communicative behaviors that they exhibit during dyadic play interactions with adults.

Differences in conversational styles during distinct types of play interactions are also found within the same cultural or socioeconomic group (Heath, 1983; Laosa, 1982). For example, Jackson-Maldonado (1994) compared the free-play language behavior of children and parents who were from very low socioeconomic backgrounds in two different play contexts. As in the literature, the mothers were asked to play with their children as they would at home and were provided with a set of colorful plastic toys like those typically used in child language research. The mothers had two reactions to these requests, both of which have a strong effect on the validity of the samples collected using the language-sampling technique. First, many of the mothers stated that they did not play with their children at home. Thus, the interactional context that was provided for the mother–child dyad was not a natural one and was unlikely to provide a typical sample of the child's language. Second, the mothers typically did not allow their children to play with the colorful toys during the language sampling sessions, saying *"No lo toques"* [Don't touch it] when the children tried to do so. Presumably, the mothers were afraid of having their children break these attractive toys that belonged to the experimenter. When presented with common household objects found in the market, such as clay pots, wooden spoons, *molcajetes* [stone hand grinders], and fruit or vegetable forms made from natural materials, however, the mothers eagerly encouraged the children to play with these objects (Carrillo Aranguren, Jackson-Maldonado, Thal, & Flores, 1997; Jackson-Maldonado, 1997).

Parent Report

Parent report is a component of many widely used screening tools that have been developed for English-speaking infants and toddlers. Examples include the Birth to Three Developmental Scale (Bangs & Dodson, 1979), the Brigance Inventory of Early Development–Revised (Brigance, 1991), the Receptive-Expressive Emergent Language Test–2 (Bzoch & League, 1991), Denver II (Frankenburg et al., 1992), and the Rossetti Infant-Toddler Language Scale (Rossetti, 1995). Parent report is also incorporated into many structured assessments, such as the Sequenced Inventory of Communicative Development–Revised Edition (Hedrick, Prather, & Tobin, 1984) and the PLS-3 (Zimmerman et al., 1993a).

Instruments such as the CDIs (Fenson et al., 1992/1993; Fenson et al., 2000) and the Language Development Survey (Rescorla, 1989) that are stand-alone parent report instruments have been developed and are now widely used with infants and toddlers who speak a number of languages (including English, Italian, and Finnish, to name a few). The adaptation of the CDIs to Spanish provides the tools for the use of the parent report technique with Spanish-speaking infants and toddlers as well. Using an early version of the Inventarios with Mexican and Mexican American children, Jackson-Maldonado, Thal, Marchman, Bates, and Gutierrez-Clellen (1993) found that parent report provided valid assessments of early language development in the 8- to 30-month age range. This finding has been confirmed with additional studies (Thal, Jackson-Maldonado, & Acosta, 2000) using revised versions of the Inventarios. Importantly, parent report has been found to demonstrate good validity in assessments of language skills in bilingual Spanish- and English-speaking children, as well (Marchman & Martínez-Sussmann, 2002; Patterson, 1998, 2000). (For more information, see the section in Chapter 4 called "Validity of the Inventarios.")

The oldest type of parent report is the diary. Parent diaries have a long and respectable history in developmental psycholinguistics (e.g., Dromi, 1987; Leopold, 1949; Stern & Stern, 1907; Tomasello, 1992), particularly in the Spanish-speaking world (Alarcos Llorach, 1976; Hernández Pina, 1984; López Ornat,

1988; Truex, 1982). Most experts in this field recognize that this form of parent report constitutes an invaluable source of information about the child's day-to-day progress in the early stages of language development. Most diary studies, however, have been published by parent-scientists who have had extensive training in the observation of language behavior, training that the average parent lacks. Nonetheless, the average parent is quite adept at observing his or her child's behavior. Modern-day parent report instruments have therefore been designed to capture the advantages of the diary study method in a user-friendly format.

Parent report has a number of inherent advantages over other means of assessing child language. First, it can provide data that are more representative of infant and toddler language than laboratory samples because the parent has the opportunity to observe the child in a wide range of situations. Second, parent report may be less influenced by performance factors, such as word frequency, than is direct clinic or laboratory observation (Fenson et al., 1992/1993). As Bates, Bretherton, and Snyder have emphasized, parent report reflects "what the child knows," whereas observations at home or in the laboratory are better assessments of "what the child prefers to use" (1988, p. 96). Third, parent report is a cost-effective means for a rapid general evaluation of language that can be valuable for screening purposes in clinical and educational settings as well as research applications. Fourth, parent report can be obtained in advance of actually seeing a child and, therefore, can help in selecting assessment procedures for more in-depth analyses. Clinicians can also use parent report as an adjunct to assess the representativeness of their own evaluations. Finally, because parent report is based on behavior in contexts outside the clinic or laboratory, it is especially valuable in monitoring changes in language over time. Therefore, this technique may be particularly useful for monitoring the progress of intervention.

Of course, parent report is not without its limitations as a means to assess language abilities (Feldman et al., 2000; Fenson, Bates, et al., 2000; Tomasello & Mervis, 1994). Parents may be accused of being biased observers, tending to either under- or overestimate their child's developing abilities. To combat these potential limitations, Fenson and colleagues (1992/1993) argued that parent report is most likely to be accurate under two conditions: when assessment is limited to current and emergent behaviors and when a recognition format is used. Each of these conditions places fewer demands on the respondent's memory, relative to retrospective reports and/or "free-form" reports. The recognition strategy capitalizes on the greater ease of picking out possible examples from a set, as contrasted with recalling those examples anew. That is, it is better to ask parents to report on their child's vocabulary by selecting words from a comprehensive or representative list rather than to have them write down all of the words they can recall hearing their child use. The recognition format also reduces the need for parents to make inferences about the nature of the questions being asked and/or their child's level of ability relative to other children (e.g., "What do they mean by animal words?" "What do they mean by 'lots' of animal words?").

SCOPE AND DESCRIPTION OF THE INVENTARIOS

Like the CDIs in English, the Inventarios are stand-alone parent report instruments that are designed to approximate the value of good parent diaries and to minimize the well-known limitations of parent report. In particular, the Inventarios target current and emerging behaviors, rely on recognition memory, and avoid retrospective accounts. These instruments are easy to administer and interpret and allow collection of data on a relatively large scale. The general effectiveness of these instruments, in terms of their reliability and validity in the assessment of key language milestones, is documented in more detail in the sections in Chapter 4 called "Reliability of the Inventarios" and "Validity of the Inventarios."

As with the English CDIs, the goal of the Inventarios is to yield reliable information on the course of language development from a child's early signs of comprehension, to his or her first nonverbal gestural signals, to the expansion of early vocabulary, to the beginnings of grammar. The structure of the Inventarios closely follows the English CDIs in organization and content, including two separate forms designed for different age ranges.

Inventario I is designed for use with 8- to 18-month-old typically developing children (see the section in Chapter 3 called "Evaluation of Older Children with Language Delay" for information about using Inventario I with older children who may have delays in language development). Those users who are familiar with the English CDIs will note that Inventario I extends the upper age limit of the English CDI: Words and Gestures by 2 months, enabling the assessment of receptive vocabulary and gesture use in children up to 18 months of age. This was done because few ceiling effects were observed in the English CDI at 16 months on key variables or in preliminary studies with the Inventarios. Inventario II is designed for children from 16 to 30 months of age, identical to the age range that is appropriate for the English CDI: Words and Sentences.

Primeras Palabras y Gestos (Inventario I)

Inventario I is composed of two major parts (see Table 1.1). *I[a] Parte: Primeras Palabras* [Part I: Early Words], begins with three short subsections. Section A, *Comprensión Temprana* [First Signs of Understanding] includes three questions designed to determine whether the child has begun to respond to language at all. In Section B, *Comprensión de las Primeras Frases* [Phrases Understood], the parent chooses the phrases that their child understands from a 28-item list. The third section, *Maneras de Hablar* [Starting to Talk], includes two questions, one asking parents about the frequency with which the child imitates words or phrases and one asking about the frequency with which the child labels objects.

The major portion of Part I is Section D, a 428-item *Lista de Vocabulario* [Vocabulary Checklist]. Here, parents indicate which words their child *comprende* [understands] and which words their child *comprende y dice* [under-

Table 1.1. Components of *Primeras Palabras y Gestos* (Inventario I)

***Iª Parte: Primeras Palabras* [Part I: Early Words]**	
A. *Comprensión Temprana* [First Signs of Understanding]	General questions about early comprehension of familiar words and phrases (3 items)
B. *Comprensión de las Primeras Frases* [Phrases Understood]	Comprehension of everyday phrases and routines (28 items)
C. *Maneras de Hablar* [Starting to Talk]	Imitation and labeling (2 items)
D. *Lista de Vocabulario* [Vocabulary Checklist]	Classification of whether the child *comprende* [understands] or *comprende y dice* [understands and says] words in 22 categories (428 items)
***IIª Parte: Gestos y Acciones* [Part II: Actions and Gestures]**	
A. *Primeros Gestos* [First Communicative Gestures]	A through E (64 items) form the *Total de Gestos* [Total Gestures] summary score.
B. *Juegos con Adultos y Rutinas* [Games and Routines]	A and B (21 items) form the *Gestos Tempranos* [Early Gestures] summary score.
C. *Acciones con Objetos* [Actions with Objects]	C through E (43 items) form the *Gestos Tardíos* [Later Gestures] summary score.
D. *Jugar a Ser Adulto* [Pretending to Be a Parent]	
E. *Imitación de Otros Tipos de Actividades de Adultos* [Imitating Other Adult Actions]	

stands and says]. Inventario I targets both vocabulary comprehension and production in this age range because information about comprehension vocabulary is particularly important during those months when spoken language is still minimal. In addition, longitudinal studies of infants and toddlers in other languages have suggested that language comprehension is a better predictor of later language development (Bates et al., 1988) and of persistent language impairment than is language production during the early stages of development (for a review, see Thal & Katich, 1996). A category of use without understanding was not included because, as Fenson et al. (1992/1993) have pointed out, it is not clear whether parents can or cannot reliably distinguish between words that children use with and without understanding.

The *Lista de Vocabulario* is organized into 22 semantic categories. Ten of the categories contain nouns (*Animales* [Animals], *Vehículos* [Vehicles], *Alimentos y Bebidas* [Food and Drink], *Ropa* [Clothing], *Partes del Cuerpo* [Body Parts], *Juguetes* [Toys], *Utensilios de la Casa* [Small Household Items], *Muebles y Cuartos* [Furniture and Rooms], *Lugares y Objetos Fuera de la Casa* [Outside Things and Places to Go], and *Personas* [People]). Additional sections include words in the following categories: *Sonidos de Cosas y Animales* [Sound Effects and Animal Sounds]; *Rutina Diaria, Reglas Sociales y Juegos* [Games and Routines]; *Acciones y Procesos (Verbos)* [Action Words (Verbs)]; *Estados* [*State Verbs]; *Tiempo* [Words About Time]; *Cualidades y Atributos* [Descriptive Words]; *Pronombres* [Pronouns], *Preguntas* [Question Words]; *Artículos* [*Articles]; *Cuantificadores y Adverbios* [Quantifiers]; *Locativos* [*Locatives]; and *Preposiciones* [*Prepositions]. In *Acciones y Procesos (Verbos)* [Action Words (Verbs)] and *Estados* [*State Verbs], verbs are presented in the infinitive form. Parents, however, should be told that a word should be marked as *comprende* [understands] or *comprende y dice* [understands and says] if any form is used by the child. (See the section in Chapter 2 called "Administering the Inventarios" and Appendices B and C for more instructions to parents.)

The second part of Inventario I, *II^a Parte: Gestos y Acciones* [Part II: Actions and Gestures] focuses on children's use of communicative and symbolic gestures. This section offers an opportunity for appraisal of a range of early communicative and representational skills that are not dependent on verbal expression. Gestures have been shown to play an important role in an infant's early developing communicative skills (Bates, Benigni, Bretherton, Camaioni, & Volterra, 1979; Caselli, 1990). Research has also revealed that gestures may serve as an index of early symbolic skill and as a cornerstone of linguistic development (Acredolo & Goodwyn, 1985, 1988; Bates et al., 1979; Bates et al., 1988; Butterworth & Morissette, 1996; Capirci, Iverson, Pizzutto, & Volterra, 1996; Goldin-Meadow & Morford, 1985; Iverson, Capirci, & Caselli, 1994; Pérez & Castro, 1988; Piaget, 1962; Thal & Bates, 1988; Thal & Tobias, 1992, 1994; Thal, Tobias, & Morrison, 1991). This section complements the linguistic items indexed in Part I and may be especially useful for assessing communicative and symbolic skills in infants who have little expressive language and in children who are demonstrating signs of language delay or impairment (Terrell & Schwartz, 1988; Terrell, Schwartz, Prelock, & Messick 1984; Thal & Tobias, 1992, 1994; Thal, Tobias, et al., 1991).

The 64 gestures are organized into five categories. The items in Section A, *Primeros Gestos* [First Communicative Gestures], signal the onset of intentional communication, an important prerequisite for language. These include the deictic gestures of giving, showing, pointing, and reaching and a number of conventionalized communicative gestures (e.g., shaking the head "no"). Often, these early gestures are combined with vocalizations in making requests or in drawing an adult's attention to something (e.g., Bates et al., 1979; Pérez & Castro, 1988; Rollins & Snow, 1998). The items in Section B, *Juegos con Adultos y Rutinas* [Games and Routines], form an important part of the early social interactive basis for communicative development (Bruner, 1977). The most common items in Sections A and B typically are seen in a majority of children well before the end of the first year of life (Bates et al., 1979; Bates, Camaioni, & Volterra, 1975; Locke, 1978). Results from a number of studies of preverbal development suggest that the gestures in Section A are strongly predictive of the emergence of meaningful speech (Bates et al., 1979; Thal & Bates, 1988). For example, many children nod or shake their head before they use the words "yes" and "no" or reach for an object to request it before they use the object's name to request it. The predictive value of the gestures in Section B is less well known, although there is evidence that children's participation in social games and routines has a key role in the regulation and maintenance of joint attention (Rollins & Snow, 1998; Tomasello & Farrar, 1986). Taken together, the items in Sections A and B compose the summary score called *Gestos Tempranos* [Early Gestures].

The child's use of gestures such as those in Section C, *Acciones con Objetos* [Actions with Objects], and Section E, *Imitación de Otros Tipos de Actividades de Adultos* [Imitating Other Adult Actions], expresses a growing understanding of the world of objects and the uses of things (Bretherton, 1984; Piaget, 1952). The child's appropriate use of objects distinguishes these actions from the earlier undifferentiated responses of the younger infant and signals an emerging representational capacity (Fenson, Kagan, Kearsley, & Zelazo, 1976). The items in Section D, *Jugar a Ser Adulto* [Pretending to Be a Parent], are among the first types of true symbolic gestures, preceded only by similar actions directed toward the self (Piaget, 1962). These types of actions generally emerge a few months later in the child's spontaneous play than the accommodative acts in Sections C and E (Fenson & Ramsay, 1980). The sum of responses in Sections C, D, and E represents *Gestos Tardíos* [Later Gestures].

During the norming studies, a final section of Inventario I, Section F, *Acciones con un Objeto en Vez de Otro* [Pretend Objects], asked parents whether their child has begun to pretend that one object is another one during play and, if so, to write an example. A similar section appeared on the CDI. In the norming studies of both the English CDIs and the Spanish Inventarios, however, results for this section were highly unstable. As a result, this section was not included in this edition of the Inventarios and will be deleted from the next edition of the CDIs.

Palabras y Enunciados (Inventario II)

Inventario II is designed for use with children between 16 and 30 months of age and assesses various aspects of the acquisition of vocabulary and grammar. The general format is similar to Inventario I; however, there are several age-related differences (see Table 1.2). *Iª Parte: El Uso de Palabras* [Part I: Words Children Use], contains a 680-word vocabulary checklist. In contrast to the checklist on Inventario I, the *Lista de Vocabulario* [Vocabulary Checklist] on Inventario II is limited to language production, asking parents to only indicate the words that their child *dice* [says]. This is due to the fact that parents are less likely to be able to keep track of both comprehension and production as their child's expressive language begins to grow rapidly toward the end of the second year of life. In addition, Inventario II has a greater number of words than Inventario I because of expected age-related increases in vocabulary.

The *Lista de Vocabulario* is organized into 23 semantic categories. In general, these categories directly parallel those included on the vocabulary checklist on Inventario I. Eleven of these categories contain only nouns—*Animales* [Animals], *Vehículos* [Vehicles], *Alimentos y Bebidas* [Food and Drink], *Ropa* [Clothing], *Partes del Cuerpo* [Body Parts], *Juguetes* [Toys], *Utensilios de la Casa* [Small Household Items], *Muebles y Cuartos* [Furniture and Rooms], *Objetos Fuera de la Casa* [Outside Things], *Lugares Fuera de la Casa* [Places to Go], and *Personas* [People]). Additional categories include *Sonidos de Cosas y Animales* [Sound Effects and Animal Sounds], *Rutina Diaria, Reglas Sociales y Juegos* [Games and Routines], *Acciones y Procesos (Verbos)* [Action Words], *Estados* [*State Verbs], *Cualidades y Atributos* [Descriptive Words], *Tiempo* [Words About Time], *Pronombres y Modificadores* [Pronouns], and *Preguntas* [Question Words]. A *Conectivos* [Connecting Words] category was also included on Inventario II because some children between 16 and 30 months of age use multiword utterances that include connectives. Items in the *Preposiciones*

Table 1.2. Components of *Palabras y Enunciados* (Inventario II)

***Iª Parte: El Uso de Palabras* [Part I: Words Children Use]**	
A. *Lista de Vocabulario* [Vocabulary Checklist]	Classification of whether the child *dice* [says] words in 23 semantic categories (680 items)
B. *Cómo Usa y Comprende el Niño/a el Lenguaje* [How Children Use Words]	Use of language to refer to past, future, and absent objects and people (5 items)
***IIª Parte: Oraciones y Gramática* [Part II: Sentences and Grammar]**	
A. *Formas de Verbos* [*Verb Forms]	Present indicative verb conjugations (regular *-ar, -ir, -er* verb types) (12 items)
	Preterit (past tense) verb conjugations (regular *-ar, -ir, -er* verb types) (6 items)
	Imperative verb conjugations (regular *-ar, -ir, -er* verb types) (6 items)
Combinación de Palabras [Combining]	Asks whether the child has begun to combine words yet (1 item)
B. *Ejemplos* [Examples]	Space provided for three of the longest sentences the parent has heard the child say recently (basis for *M3L-Palabras* [M3L-*Words])
C. *Complejidad de Frases* [Complexity]	Sentence pairs that contrast in length and grammatical complexity (37 item pairs); asks which form is most like the way the child currently talks

y Artículos and *Cuantificadores y Adverbios* sections correspond roughly to items in the Prepositions and Locations and the Quantifiers and Articles sections on the English CDI: Words and Sentences. Users of both Inventario I and Inventario II should notice that *Preposiciones* [Prepositions] and *Artículos* [Articles], which are separate sections on Inventario I, are combined into one section on Inventario II, whereas *Lugares y Objetos Fuera de la Casa* [Outside Things and Places to Go], which is one section on Inventario I, is divided into two sections on Inventario II.

During the period from 16 to 30 months of age, language use is also characterized by first word combinations, emerging syntax, and increasingly complex use of morphological forms. In order to capture this developmental information, *IIª Parte: Oraciones y Gramática* [Part II: Sentences and Grammar] of Inventario II is devoted to the assessment of several aspects of morphology and syntax. Section A, *Formas de Verbos* [*Verb Forms], asks parents to indicate their child's production of three common regular verbs (one in each of the three major verb-ending classes, *-ar, -er,* and *-ir*). These verbs are listed in selected conjugations in three categories: Presente [*Present] (12 items), Pasado [*Past] (6 items), and Imperativo [*Imperative] (6 items). These tenses were chosen because studies of Spanish language acquisition have shown these to be among the most frequent and earliest tense forms to appear (Aguado Alonso, 1989; Anderson, 1995; Bedore, 1999, 2001; Beléndez-Soltero, 1980; Dato, 1975; Fernández Martínez, 1994; Gathercole, Sebastián, & Soto, 1999; González, 1983; Hernández Pina, 1984; Jackson-Maldonado & Maldonado, 2001; Maez, 1983; Merino & Spencer, 1983).

In the second part of Section A, parents are asked whether the child has begun to produce word combinations in the following way: *¿Su hijo/a ya* *empezó a combinar palabras, como 'papá coche' o 'más agua'?* [Has your child begun to combine words like "daddy car" or "more water"?]. (This part of Inventario II is hereafter referred to as *Combinación de Palabras* [Combining].) If parents indicate *todavía no* [not yet], they are told to stop at that point and to not complete the subsequent Sections B and C.

In Section B, *Ejemplos* [Examples], parents are asked to provide examples of their child's "best" early utterances. Similar to the English CDI, Section B asks the parents to write examples of the three longest utterances that they have recently heard their child say. This method is based on the work of Rescorla (1989) and has been used in other versions of the CDIs. These example sentences yield an index of morphosyntax that is strongly correlated with mean length of utterance from spontaneous language samples in English (Dale, 1991) and in Spanish (Thal et al., 2000). (See the section in Chapter 4 called "Validity of the Inventarios" for more information.) Section B is included so that clinicians and researchers can have an additional index of toddler speech that is based on the child's actual utterances.

On Inventario II, mean length of the three longest utterances is calculated by computing the average number of words in the example sentences provided by the parent, yielding *M3L-Palabras* [M3L-*Words]. This contrasts with the computation in morphemes, as is typically done in analyses of English child language data. The calculation of *M3L-Palabras* [M3L-*Words] adheres to procedures most commonly used in the study of acquisition of Romance languages (Aguado Alonso, 1989; Anderson, 1995; Echeverría, 1979; Gutiérrez-Clellen, Restrepo, Bedore, Peña, & Anderson, 2000; Schnell de Acedo, 1994). As Anderson (1995) and Gutiérrez-Clellen et al. (2000) noted, there are two important reasons for choosing to use words rather than morphemes when calculating utterance length in Spanish. First, because no specific criteria have been established for counting morphemes in Spanish, there is considerable variation across studies (García, 1978; Gutiérrez-Clellen et al., 2000; Kvaal, Shipstead-Cox, Nevitt, Hodson, & Launer, 1988; Linares-Orama & Sanders, 1977; Maez, 1983). Second, mean length of utterance in morphemes was established for use with English, a language that has limited morphology. Although it works well as a general measure of grammatical level in English, there is good reason to believe that it will not work in the same way in languages with very rich grammatical morphology (Anderson, 1995; Gutiérrez-Clellen et al., 2000). See Appendix E for more detailed instructions regarding the transcription and scoring of example utterances.

In Section C, *Complejidad de Frases* [Complexity], parents are asked to choose which member of each of 37 phrase/sentence pairs best reflects the way their child talks. In each case, the second member of each pair is the more advanced form. To provide an adequate developmental range, items were selected from a number of sources in which spontaneous language samples were described. These included data from Castilian Spanish (Hernández Pina, 1984; López Ornat, Fernández, Gallo, & Mariscal, 1994), samples of Spanish-speaking children growing up in the United States (Kvaal et al., 1988; Maez, 1983), doctoral dissertations (Jackson, 1989), and transcripts of children living in Mexico collected by the first author of this manual (Jackson-Maldonado, 1984). Use of some unpublished sources was necessary because of the scarcity of published studies of Mexican Spanish language acquisition when the Inventarios were being developed. Pairs of phrases were constructed by using one example from the language samples and basing the counterpart on similar structures observed in the samples. In some cases, the example from the language sample was the more complex phrase and a simpler form was constructed. In other cases, the example from the language sample was the simpler form and a more complex phrase was constructed using transcript examples of possible structures (see Thal et al., 2000, and Appendix F for a description of Section C). Pairs increase in complexity from telegraphic-like phrases with noncanonical word order to inflected verbs and nouns and canonical word order (first 10 pairs); from shorter to longer phrases with function words (pairs 11–20); to inflected and more complex verb and prepositional phrases (pairs 21–30); and, finally, adding complexity with connectives in the last 7 phrase pairs.

2

ADMINISTRATION, SCORING, AND INTERPRETATION

The administration of the Inventarios and the *Forma de Información Básica* [Basic Information Form] (Appendix A) is designed to be self-explanatory. *Nevertheless, researchers and clinicians (and relevant staff) who plan to use the Inventarios are strongly encouraged to become thoroughly familiar with the guidelines for their administration.* We provide an overview of general administration and scoring issues in this chapter.

ADMINISTERING THE INVENTARIOS

General Instructions

Written instructions are provided at the beginning of each section of the Inventarios. Even though written instructions are available to a parent, it is not always customary in the Hispanic culture to read them. Therefore, the examiner may wish to explain the instructions verbally to parents and/or provide an additional handout that outlines important points. Basic points for parents to remember, along with tips for the examiner in italic type, are laid out next. Example handouts (in English and Spanish) that summarize the general instructions are provided in Appendix B.

- Indicate ***Fecha de nacimiento*** **[Birthdate]** and ***Fecha de hoy*** **[Today's date]** on form.
  Parents should be shown where to indicate these dates, as they are crucial in the calculation of the age of the child at the time of administration.
- Complete ***Forma de Información Básica*** **[Basic Information Form]** (Appendix A).
  This brief questionnaire asking basic contact, demographic, and medical history information is provided in English and in Spanish in Appendix A.

- Please **read instructions** carefully!
The written instructions can be highlighted directly on the form and/or shown to the parents. When necessary, instructions may be read (or summarized) aloud for the parents and the procedures for completing specific sections may be further elaborated verbally or through an additional handout in English or in Spanish (see Appendix B).

- Make sure you **complete all of the pages** of the questionnaire.
Parents may be less likely to skip pages if they are shown the entire form ahead of time.

- For Inventario I, mark the words that your child ***comprende*** **[understands]** or ***comprende y dice*** **[understands and says].** For Inventario II, mark the words that your child ***dice*** **[says].**
It is helpful to highlight the Lista de Vocabulario *[Vocabulary Checklist] and to outline the difference between* comprende *[understands] and* comprende y dice *[understands and says].*

- Do not mark **imitations.**
It is of utmost importance that parents realize that they should not attempt to test the child's ability to imitate a word or gesture. Rather, they should mark only words that the child uses spontaneously, without a direct model. If possible, it can be suggested that the parents fill out the questionnaire during a quiet time away from the child, such as during naptime.

- Give the child credit for **mispronounced** or **child words** (e.g., *pato* instead of *zapato*).
Parents should be reminded that children sometimes have their own "special" words for things or people in their family. These words are acceptable substitutes for words provided on Lista de Vocabulario *[Vocabulary Checklist].*

- Mark **words with the same meaning** as what your child understands or says (e.g., *super* for *tienda*). Take into account **names of people** (e.g., *tita* for *abuela*) or **words that are specific to your dialect/region**.
Instead of the word on Lista de Vocabulario *[Vocabulary Checklist], a child may use a different word that has the same meaning. These words may be particular to the family or to the local area in which the family currently or previously resides. Researchers and clinicians should be familiar with possible variants of the words on the* Lista de Vocabulario *[Vocabulary Checklist] and highlight those for parents when appropriate (see also Appendix C).*

- Take into account **other verb forms** (e.g., mark *dormir* if your child says *duerme*).
Many parents may not make the connection between the infinitive form provided on the Inventarios and the conjugated forms that the child may actually understand and/or produce. See Appendix C for a list of relevant conjugated forms.

- **Ask others** (e.g., other family members, nanny, child care providers) to help you fill out this form.
In many cases, one parent may only have access to a portion of the situations in which the child's language abilities are demonstrated, such as when that child is attending a child care center. It may be appropriate to ask multiple individuals to complete the forms (e.g., mother and grandmother). We suggest that parents note the names of all individuals who completed the forms on the front cover of the Inventario.
- Please use a **No. 2 pencil** to fill in the bubbles.
The use of a No. 2 pencil is necessary only if the forms are machine scored using Optical Mark Reading (OMR) machine scoring. (For more information about machine scoring, see the section in this chapter called "Automating the Scoring Process.")

Other Administration Considerations

Further review or elaboration of these basic instructions may be necessary in order to ensure that the parent understands the instructions and/or to provide specific clarifications about particular issues or sections, such as *Acciones y Procesos (Verbos)* [Action Words (Verbs)]. For more detailed explanations and additional examples, refer to Appendix C.

Parents who have low literacy levels may have difficulty or may feel apprehensive about reading and completing the forms. If this is the case, it may be best for the examiner to fill out the form together with the parents. This can be done in person or over the telephone. If families use a different dialect of Spanish, refer to Appendix C for a nonexhaustive list of word substitutes.

An additional concern arises when using the Inventarios in conjunction with the English CDIs (e.g., in assessments of children who are learning both English and Spanish). In these cases, it is particularly important to query the parents regarding their proficiency in either Spanish or English prior to their completion of the forms. In some cases, one parent may not have the language skill to complete both the Inventario and the CDI. For example, in a bilingual household in which the mother speaks primarily English but the father primarily speaks Spanish, it would not be appropriate for the mother to complete both the English CDI and the Spanish Inventarios. Again, we suggest that parents indicate who completed each form on the cover.

Finally, it is strongly recommended that the Inventarios be checked immediately upon receipt for completeness and potential inconsistencies across sections. Follow-up contacts may be necessary to fill in missing portions of the Inventarios. For example, a parent may indicate that the child combines words *de vez en cuando* [sometimes] or *muchas veces* [often] but then may not provide *Ejemplos* [Examples]. Furthermore, it may be necessary to probe for accuracy if the information provided on the form is strikingly inconsistent with age-based expectations (e.g., parents report that their 30-month-old produces only 10 words; parents report that their 12-month-old produces 300 words).

Table 2.1. Scoring Inventario I

Section of Inventario	How to score
***Iª Parte: Primeras Palabras* [Part I: First Words]**	
A. *Comprensión Temprana* [First Signs of Understanding]	For each of 3 items, record *sí* [yes] or *no* [no] responses. Add the number of *sí* [yes] responses to obtain the child's total score.
B. *Comprensión de las Primeras Frases* [Phrases Understood]	Count and record the number of *comprende* [understands] responses across all 28 items.
C. *Maneras de Hablar* [Starting to Talk]	For both items, record *de vez en cuando* [sometimes] and *muchas veces* [often] responses as *sí* [yes]. Record *todavía no* [not yet] responses as *no* [no].
D. *Lista de Vocabulario* [Vocabulary Checklist]	Count the number of responses in each subsection (22 subsections, 428 items total). Obtain the totals for *comprende* [understands] and *comprende y dice* [understands and says] separately. If both are marked for an item, count as if the parent had marked *comprende y dice* [understands and says] only. Items left blank are not counted. *To compute summary scores:* • *Comprensión de Palabras* [Words Understood]: Sum and record the number of *comprende* [understands] and *comprende y dice* [understands and says] responses across all 22 categories (428 maximum). *Note: Comprensión de Palabras* [Words Understood] will always be either equal to or greater than *Producción de Palabras* [Words Produced]. • *Producción de Palabras* [Words Produced]: Sum and record the number of *comprende y dice* [understands and says] responses in all 22 categories (428 maximum). *Note*: This score will not be greater than the *Comprensión de Palabras* [Words Understood] but may equal it.
***IIª Parte: Gestos y Acciones* [Part II: Gestures and Actions]**	
A. *Primeros Gestos* [First Communicative Gestures]	Count the number of *de vez en cuando* [sometimes] and *muchas veces* [often] responses as *sí* [yes] (13 items total). If both *de vez en cuando* [sometimes] and *muchas veces* [often] are marked for an item, include the item in the count. Treat items left blank as *todavía no* [not yet].
B. *Juegos con Adultos y Rutinas* [Games and Routines] C. *Acciones con Objetos* [Actions with Objects] D. *Jugar a Ser Adulto* [Pretending to Be a Parent] E. *Imitación de Otros Tipos de Actividades de Adultos* [Imitating Other Adult Actions]	Count the number of *sí* [yes] responses in each section (51 items total). Treat items left blank as *no* [no].
To compute summary scores: • *Total de Gestos* [Total Gestures]: Sum and record the number of *sí* [yes] responses in Sections A through E (64 maximum). • *Gestos Tempranos* [Early Gestures]: Sum and record the number of *sí* [yes] responses in Sections A and B (21 maximum). • *Gestos Tardíos* [Later Gestures]: Sum and record the number of *sí* [yes] responses in Sections C through E (43 maximum).	

Probes should be as neutral and nonthreatening as possible and should seek to clarify whether the parent understood the instructions. For example, the examiner might ask the parent, "I see that you reported that Johnny can say *ahora.* Can you give me an example of a situation in which he might say that word?" The parent may then volunteer that the child says that word "whenever I ask him to say it." This would indicate that the parent was marking words that the child produces in imitation but does not necessarily understand or use spontaneously.

SCORING THE INVENTARIOS

Users of the Inventarios have several scoring options and computerized tools at their disposal. The Inventarios are easily scored by hand, with percentile scores computed by comparing raw totals with the values in the look-up tables provided in Chapter 5. Tables 2.1 and 2.2 give pertinent information for scoring and interpreting. The *Informe del Niño/a* [Child Report Form] (see Appendix G and the subsection in this chapter called "Using the Norms, Interpreting a Child's Score") provides a convenient way to characterize summary scores (totals) and percentile values for a given child that can be provided to the parent. These are also useful summary records for researchers, clinician, physicians, or other professionals.

Hand scoring of the Inventarios is most convenient for small numbers of forms when the objective is to obtain summary scores for the various sections of the inventories. Scoring the inventory, including looking up percentiles and

Table 2.2. Scoring Inventario II

Section of Inventario	How to score
***Iª Parte: El Uso de las Palabras* [Part I: Words Children Use]**	
A. *Lista de Vocabulario* [Vocabulary Checklist]	Count the number of responses in each subsection (23 subsections). Do not count items left blank. *To compute a summary score:* • *Producción de Palabras* [Words Produced]: Sum and record the number of *dice* [says] responses (690 maximum) across all 23 categories.
B. *Cómo Usa y Comprende el Niño/a el Lenguaje* [How Children Use Words]	For each of 5 items, record *de vez en cuando* [sometimes] and *muchas veces* [often] responses as *sí* [yes]. Record *todavía no* [not yet] responses as *no* [no]). Count items left blank as *no* [no].
***IIª Parte: Oraciones y Gramática* [Part II: Sentences and Grammar]**	
A. *Formas de Verbos* [*Verb Forms]	Count the number of responses in each subsection. Do not count items left blank. Record the number of responses by section, *Presente* [*Present] (12 items), *Pasado* [*Past] (6 items), and *Imperativo* [*Imperative] (6 items).
Combinación de Palabras [Combining]	Record *de vez en cuando* [sometimes] and *muchas veces* [often] responses as *sí* [yes]. Record *todavía no* [not yet] as *no* [no]. If the item is left blank, count the response as *no* [no].
B. *Ejemplos* [Examples]	Count and record the number of words in each example utterance (maximum of 3) provided by the parent. *To compute a summary score:* • *M3L-Palabras* [M3L-*Words]: Sum the number of words in each example; divide by 3. If fewer than three examples are provided, divide by the number of examples provided (1 or 2). If *todavía no* [not yet] is marked for *Combinación de Palabras* [Combining], score *M3L-Palabras* as 1. • More detailed guidelines for scoring *M3L-Palabras* and sample utterances are provided in Appendix E.
C. *Complejidad de Frases* [Complexity]	Count and record the number of items in which the *second* (more complex) of the two alternatives (37 maximum) is marked. If both alternatives are chosen, score as if parent chose only the second. Do not count items left blank. See Appendix F for a description of the structure of the items.

completing an *Informe del Niño/a* [Child Report Form], by hand typically requires 20–30 minutes, more or less, depending on the age and language skill of the child. Users who would like to hand score the Inventarios should purchase the desktop scannable version of the forms.

Alternatively, users may choose to use a variety of tools that automate the process of tabulating and summarizing the data on the Inventarios. Computer-based tools for use with the Inventarios have become more cost-effective and user-friendly in recent years. For example, programs such as IDHC Score (Dale, 1999) and the Scoring Program for the MacArthur Communicative Development Inventories (http://www.sci.sdsu.edu/cdi/scoringdb_p.htm; hereafter referred to as the CDI Scoring Program) interface with data from a scanner, automatically tabulate summary scores, generate *Informes del Niño/a* [Child Report Forms], and track subject/client information in a database (discussed further later in this chapter).

Regardless of the specific scoring method chosen, we suggest that all users familiarize themselves with the general process and logic of scoring the Inventarios. We provide step-by-step instructions on scoring each section in Tables 2.1 (Inventario I) and 2.2 (Inventario II). In general, scoring involves four basic steps:

1. *Count* the item responses in each section.
2. *Sum* across sections to obtain summary scores, following the instructions in Tables 1.1 and 1.2 in Chapter 1.
3. *Look up* normative values in the percentile tables provided in Chapter 5 or use information provided in the tables of descriptive statistics. (See the subsection in this chapter called "Using the Norms" for more information on using normative data.)
4. *Record* item responses, summary scores (if any), and/or percentiles on an *Informe del Niño/a* [Child Report Form] in the appropriate slots. See the section in this chapter called "Using the Norms" and the subsection called "Interpreting a Child's Score." Example templates for the *Informe del Niño/a* [Child Report Form] and examples of filled-out forms are provided in Appendix G and in Appendices D and E, respectively.

Automating the Scoring Process

The time involvement and accuracy of scoring the Inventarios can be significantly improved with the use of tools that automate some or all of the scoring process. In this section, we first review the process of machine scanning the Inventarios and then describe other tools that are available to automate the scoring process, in particular, the CDI Scoring Program. Users should note that the CDI Scoring Program does not require machine-scannable data; users may hand count the Inventarios and still automate the processes of computing summary scores, looking up percentiles, and generating reports.

Machine Scanning Machine scanning is available with original forms (not photocopies) using some type of computerized system. All machine scanning systems require a scanner connected to a computer and a software program compatible with the scanner. These systems automatically read the completed Inventario form and create a data file in ASCII format, essentially a single long row of 1s and 0s for each scanned inventory. The scanned data output can then be converted to meaningful Inventario categories (e.g., total number of words produced) with the use of a program designed for or adapted to that purpose (e.g., IDHC Score, CDI Scoring Program). If you wish, you may supplement the Inventario forms with a user-completed "header sheet" that allows additional information to be added to each child's scanned record (e.g., the child's birth date, test date).

Two types of machine scoring systems are currently available. First, a traditional OMR reader (e.g., NCS, Scantron), the kind that is commonly associated with standardized testing, preprinted forms, and No. 2 pencils, can be used. (Traditional OMR readers are now available that accept forms completed in ink or pencil.) Second, forms can be scanned using a desktop image scanner, a device that is becoming an increasingly common accompaniment to PCs. Both types of automated scoring systems require a modest to substantial investment in hardware and software, as well as an initial programming of software.

Traditional OMR scanners generally involve an investment of at least $5,000. These systems are designed specifically for the purpose of scanning large numbers of standardized forms and incorporate features intended to maximize scanning speed and accuracy. For example, these systems have the capacity to process thousands of forms per hour, to automatically feed forms into the scanner, and to simultaneously read the front and back of the page in a single pass with "dual-read heads." In our experience, traditional OMR systems are generally quite accurate and can process a completed Inventario in less than 30 seconds.

Desktop image scanners are generally a less expensive option (starting at under $100 but ranging as high as $4,000) for the machine scoring of the Inventarios. These systems, however, are considerably slower and typically require more page handling by the user (e.g., turning over the pages). The desktop-scannable forms can be completed using different colors of pen or pencil (rather than only No. 2 pencil), and when bubbles are not filled in completely, the desktop-scannable forms can be scanned with greater accuracy than traditional OMR forms. At the same time, we recommend that users of either machine scoring method frequently verify the accuracy of the scanned information and encourage respondents to fill in bubbles as completely as possible using dark marks. More expensive image scanners will give the user faster scanning rates (although not as fast as the traditional OMR readers) and often come with accessories that reduce the amount of form handling by the user (e.g., automatic form feeder). Using this system, 2–3 minutes per form are generally required to complete the scanning process.

As mentioned previously, both types of scoring systems require software (e.g., Scantools, Remark) that converts the OMR information to a data file. Most manufacturers of traditional OMR scanners bundle the form-reading software with the hardware for sale. Because desktop image scanners are used for a variety of other purposes (e.g., scanning photographs), the software necessary for reading the Inventarios is generally not sold along with the scanner hardware. Several form-reading software packages, however, are currently available that are compatible with a wide range of image scanners. We are most familiar with Remark Office OMR by Principia Products, although users may wish to explore other alternatives before making a final selection.

For both types of systems, the set-up of the OMR software involves configuring the program to read the format of the Inventarios (i.e., where the bubbles are and what order to put them in the output file). Once the scanning system has been set up, processing the forms is a clerical task, although technical advice is likely to be necessary from time to time to resolve hardware and software problems. More information regarding the template configurations for scoring the CDIs and Inventarios is available on the CDI web page (http://www.sci.sdsu.edu/cdi/scoringdb_p.htm). These templates can be used with NCS Scantools software for traditional OMR readers or with Remark Office by Principia Products for desktop scanners.

CDI Scoring Program The CDI Scoring Program is designed to facilitate the tabulation, percentile calculation, report generation, and data-tracking functions associated with the use of the English and Spanish instruments. The CDI Scoring Program runs on PCs equipped with Microsoft Windows 95, 98, or XP and Microsoft Office 97 or 2000 (with Microsoft Access, Word, and Excel). (For more information and downloads, see http://www.sci.sdsu.edu/cdi/scoringdb_p.htm.) Versions are available that process all of the versions of the English CDIs (Words and Gestures; Words and Sentences; and Short Forms: Levels I, IIA, IIB, and III) and the Spanish-language Inventarios I and II.

Data from the English and Spanish instruments can be incorporated into the CDI Scoring Program in two ways. Users who hand-score the Inventarios can input data into the CDI Scoring Program by keyboard. Users view on-screen templates that allow data entry at either the category (e.g., *Sonidos de Cosas y Animales* [Sound Effects and Animal Sounds]) or the item level. Those users who choose the machine scanning option can import scanned data that are generated by either traditional or desktop image scanner systems directly into the CDI Scoring Program. The scanned data are required to have a fixed column starting point, and each scanned form should be in a single file. (Other constraints about how the scanned data are interpreted by the program are specified more fully in the documentation; see http://www.sci.sdsu.edu/cdi/scoringdb_p.htm).

The program automates several aspects of the scoring process and provides additional data tracking and analyses tools. Specifically, the program does the following:

- It automatically calculates percentiles for key variables that are included in reports to parents or for in-house use. In addition, when the *Ejemplos* [Examples] are transcribed from Inventario II following standard conventions (see Appendix E), the program automatically computes the *M3L-Palabras* [M3L-*Words] score. Finally, the program can calculate composite vocabulary scores that reflect responses from both the English CDI and Spanish Inventarios (Pearson, Fernandez, & Oller, 1995a, 1995b; Umbel, Pearson, Fernandez, & Oller, 1992). This feature is appropriate when English CDI and Spanish Inventario data are available for a given child at (or near) the same age in months (see also Marchman & Martínez-Sussmann, 2002).

- The program generates *Informes del Niño/a* [Child Report Forms] in both English and Spanish. The program also generates a cover letter that is intended to accompany an *Informe del Niño/a.* Letter templates can be modified to meet the users' own specific needs and can be tailored for several subpopulations (e.g., a set for participants with typical language development, a set for children with delayed language development). Examples of *Informes del Niño/a* and parent letters for both the English CDI and Spanish Inventarios are available for viewing at http://www.sci.sdsu.edu/cdi/scoringdb_p.htm (click on the links in the yellow box).
- The program provides database management and tracking tools by storing CDI and Inventario data and a variety of demographic and medical information as provided on the *Forma de Información Básica* [Basic Information Form] (see Appendix A).
- The program generates summaries of data, selecting participants by any criterion and outputting any variable from the CDIs or Inventarios and/or user-defined variables. These can be output into a table (in Microsoft Access format) or a spreadsheet (in Microsoft Excel format), which can then be imported by statistical packages as needed.

Choosing a Scoring Option

Three factors should be considered when making a decision about which procedures to adopt for scoring the Inventarios: 1) the number of forms to be processed, 2) the level of data description and analyses of interest, and 3) the availability of computer support/equipment or outside scanning services and support personnel.

Number of Forms Given the necessary equipment and technical support or the possibility of using outside scanning arrangements, machine scanning is best for users who plan relatively large-scale endeavors and who plan to be regular users of the instruments. The decision whether to use machine scanning should also be made in the context of the types of data that are to be analyzed. Given the wide range of potential uses of the Inventarios, it is difficult to determine a precise number of forms for which scanning would become more expedient than hand scoring, although 150–200 would be a rough estimate. If the number of forms to be processed does not warrant the investment of machine scanning, recall that hand-scorers may automatize the computing of summary scores and percentiles and the generation of *Informes del Niño/a* [Child Report Forms] by using the CDI Scoring Program.

Types of Analyses Scanning is a particularly attractive option when the user is interested in analyses at the individual item level and at the category level. The alternative to scanning when individual item data are of interest is to enter each data point by keyboard into a computer file. Entering individual item data requires more than 900 data points per child for Inventario I, plus additional columns for designating the child's subject number, birth date, and so forth. Inventario II requires more than 700 data points. Inputting the data is a labor-intensive endeavor, even with a modest number of forms, and some data entry errors must be expected. Of course, a clinician or researcher interested in examining item data for an individual child would not need to scan forms for this purpose. A child's knowledge of specific words or types of words could be easily evaluated by hand tabulation. In addition, the required time and potential for errors is significantly reduced with the CDI Scoring Program. Here, data entry templates have prespecified slots for each item, reducing possible confusion across items. Furthermore, the program imports default values into the templates, so that only items that differ from that default value need to be entered by the user via the keyboard (e.g., enter only the *sí* [yes] responses).

Availability of Equipment and Support Personnel Machine scanning requires an investment in hardware and software that many researchers and clinicians do not have readily available. Some schools, hospitals, and universities, however, already have the equipment necessary for scanning forms using this method and, when provided with the appropriate software templates, may be able to scan inventories on a contract basis. The availability of these resources may significantly reduce the start-up costs associated with machine scanning using traditional OMR systems. As mentioned previously, desktop scanners are becoming increasingly available in many university and clinical settings. The conversion of these desktop scanners to also process CDIs and Inventarios may require the purchase and configuration of software.

Once a machine scanning system is in place, the scanning of the forms becomes a clerical task. It should be kept in mind that prior to scanning, a few minutes of preparation time are generally required for each form, to separate the pages for insertion into the scanner, copy the subject number onto each page (in case the stack of forms is ever dropped), prepare the header sheets (if appropriate), and make sure that no pages have been inadvertently skipped. If OMR scanning is used, preparation is also required before scanning each form to ensure that each response bubble is fully filled in (as opposed to being marked by a check mark or an *X*), to pencil over responses marked in ink, and to erase stray pencil marks. The preparation time may equal that required for hand scoring. Nonetheless when the individual item data are of interest, scanning is strongly recommended for data sets in excess of 50–100 inventories.

USING THE NORMS

The percentile scores provided in Chapter 5 allow establishment of the status of individual children, relative to their age-mates (with an age correction applied for children who were born prematurely), on each major section of Inventario I and Inventario II. Following Fenson et al. (1992/1993), the tabled values are "smoothed" scores derived by plotting the best-fitting linear or logistic curve through the raw percentile scores (in 5 percentile increments, e.g., 5th, 10th, 15th) for each inventory summary score. This procedure compensates for irregularities in raw scores produced by random variation.

Despite the absence of statistically reliable differences between girls and boys at the monthly intervals, the fitted curves are consistently higher for girls for most measures on both Inventario I and II. Thus, separate tables are provided for girls and for boys in Chapter 5. For most research and clinical purposes, it is recommended that percentile scores be computed on the basis of both age and sex. However, for the convenience of users who wish to score forms without reference to gender, fitted percentile tables for the sexes combined are also presented for each major scale (see Tables 5.1, 5.4, 5.7, 5.10, 5.13, 5.16, 5.19, 5.22, and 5.25). For the Inventario I sections *Comprensión Temprana* [First Signs of Understanding] and *Maneras de Hablar* [Starting to Talk] and the Inventario II sections *Cómo Usa y Comprende el Niño/a el Lenguaje* [How Children Use Words], and *Combinación de Palabras* [Combining], scores are presented in tables that show the percentage of children reported to use the relevant form of language (see Tables 4.6, 4.9, 4.20, and 4.23, respectively, in Chapter 4), rather than in tables that show percentiles.

In all cases, caution should be exercised when applying the norms to children from families in which the parents have very low education and socioeconomic levels and to children whose chronological ages exceed the upper limits of the inventories. (See the section in this chapter called "Using the Norms with Children from Families of Low Socioeconomic Status" and the section in Chapter 3 called "Evaluation of Older Children with Language Delay.")

Interpreting a Child's Score

Percentile rank tables provide a convenient method for identifying where an individual child falls within a group. Percentile values can be derived from the look-up tables (see Chapter 5) or generated automatically with the CDI Scoring Program. We outline the general instructions for determining percentile ranks and percentage distributions. These instructions are particularly useful for those who score and derive percentile equivalences by hand; however, we recommend that all users familiarize themselves with the logic of the process, even if automated procedures are applied.

1. Determine responses or summary scores using the guidelines in Tables 2.1 (Inventario I) and 2.2 (Inventario II) (e.g., *Comprensión de Palabras* [Words Understood], *Producción de Palabras* [Words Produced]).
2. Find the table that corresponds to the subscale for the child's gender (e.g., Table 5.5 for *Comprensión de Palabras* [Words Understood] for girls on Inventario I, Table 5.21 for *Producción de Palabras* [Words Produced] for boys on Inventario II).

3. Go down the column of the child's age until you find the number closest to the raw score for the child.

4. Cross over to the far left of that row to obtain the percentile equivalence. If the child's score corresponds *exactly* to a number in the table, assign that exact percentile equivalence score. For example, a 13-month-old girl who is reported to comprehend 44 words falls at the 20th percentile; in other words, 20 percent of the girls in the norming sample at 13 months of age had a vocabulary comprehension score that was at or below 44 words. A 14-month-old girl reported to understand 123 words would have a percentile score of 50th (i.e., the score falls at the middle of the distribution for that month). A girl of the same age with a score of 275 would fall at the 90th percentile, meaning that she is in the top 10% of her age group.

   If the child's score falls *between* two numbers in the table, there are two ways to assign a percentile equivalence value. It is reasonable to use the conservative strategy of giving the percentile that is below the real score. For example, if a 13-month-old girl were reported to comprehend 38 words, that score would fall between the 15th (34 words) and the 20th (44 words) percentiles. Conservatively, she would be placed at the 15th percentile. The most accurate method, however, is to interpolate and assign an exact percentile. To interpolate, subtract the low from the high numbers in the table to get the range in raw scores between the two percentile values (e.g., 44 – 34 = 10; 10 words is the difference between the 15th and 20th percentiles). Divide that difference by 5 to compute the raw score that reflects a 1-percentile unit change, in this case 2 words (10 ÷ 5). Add this number to the lower score in the range until the child's actual score is reached. In this case, the girl would be placed at the 17th percentile (34 words = 15th percentile; 36 words = 16th percentile; 38 words = 17th percentile). (*Note:* The CDI Scoring Program automatically computes exact percentile values using a similar interpolation procedure.)

   In some cases, the same raw score is represented by a *range* of percentile scores. In this case, assign the higher percentile. For example, if a 15-month-old girl were reported to comprehend 6 words, her score would correspond to both the 25th and the 30th percentiles (because they are both 6 words). She should be placed at the 30th percentile.

5. For sections for which full percentile tables are not available, use the tables that present the distributions of children by age in order to estimate how the child compares with other children of the same age. For example, Table 4.23 shows the percentage of children at each age with *sí* [yes] responses on *Combinación de Palabras* [Combining]. (*Note:* As mentioned in Table 2.2, *sí* [yes] responses represent the sum of *de vez en cuando* [sometimes] and *muchas veces* [often] responses). A 28-month-old boy whose parents report that he is not combining words falls in the lowest 11.6% of 28-month-old boys in the norming sample, given that 88.4% of the boys at this age were reported to combine words. Table 4.20 shows the distribution of *sí* [yes] responses on *Cómo Usa y Comprende el Niño/a el Lenguaje* [How Chil-

dren Use Words]. A 20-month-old child whose parent reports that he or she does not talk about absent objects falls in the lowest 15.1% of children her or his age (84.9% of 20-month-old children do refer to absent objects). If the parent were to report instead that the child talks about events that occurred in the past, the child would be placed in the upper 29% of the children in the norming sample (71% of 20-month-old children in the sample did not use the past tense).

Additional Considerations In evaluating percentile scores, it is important to examine the distribution of the raw scores at that age. For ages at which the skills in question are just emerging, very small differences in raw scores can sometimes produce large shifts in percentile scores. As may be seen in Table 5.9 in Chapter 5, for example, the entire range in scores for *Producción de Palabras* [Words Produced] is 20 words (0–20) for 8-month-old boys. For a 12-month-old boy, a difference of 10 words (0 versus 10) would put him at or between the 35th and the 75th percentiles. As shown in Table 5.21, this same range in raw scores would fall within a single 5-percentile increment for a 27-month-old boy. Vocabulary production presents the most extreme instances of this nature, but there are several other measures for which a restricted range in raw scores when a skill is just emerging creates unstable percentile levels. Caution must be exercised when using these scales.

Interpreting Inventario I

Three major features of communicative development can be derived from Inventario I: comprehension of words and phrases, production of words, and production of actions and gestures. Inventario I also includes two other sections (*Comprensión Temprana* [First Signs of Understanding], and *Maneras de Hablar* [Starting to Talk]) that do not provide percentile scores. Specific instructions for interpreting the data on Inventario I are provided in Table 2.3.

Interpreting Inventario II

Inventario II contains eight sections. Three sections yield percentile scores: *Lista de Vocabulario* [Vocabulary], *M3L-Palabras* [M3L-*Words], and *Complejidad de Frases* [Complexity]. In developing profiles for individual children, the examiner can also make use of scores on *Cómo Usa y Comprende el Niño/a el Lenguaje* [How Children Use Words], *Formas de Verbos* [*Verb Forms], and *Combinación de Palabras* [Combining] by consulting the percentage distribution tables in Chapter 4 (see Tables 4.20–4.23). Specific instructions for interpreting the data on Inventario II are provided in Table 2.4. Appendix E provides detailed information about how *M3L-Palabras* [M3L-*Words] is calculated.

Using the Norms with Children from Families of Low Socioeconomic Status

The children in the normative sample for the Inventarios were from several areas in the states of Guanajuato, Querétaro, and Sinaloa, Mexico. The effect of

Table 2.3. Interpreting a child's score on Inventario I

Section of Inventario	Descriptive statistics/ developmental trends	Percentile tables	Comments
***Iª Parte: Primeras Palabras* [Part I: Early Words]**			
A. *Comprensión Temprana* [First Signs of Understanding]	Table 4.6	—	For each of 3 items, compare response totals with percentage of children with that number of *sí* [yes] reponses at that child's age.
B. *Comprensión de las Primeras Frases* [Phrases Understood]	Tables 4.7 and 4.8; Figures 4.1 and 4.2	Tables 5.1–5.3	Use percentile tables for *Comprensión de las Primeras Frases* [Phrases Understood] (28 items).
C. *Maneras de Hablar* [Starting to Talk]	Table 4.9; Figure 4.3	—	For each of 2 items, compare responses with percentage of children with that number of *sí* [yes] responses at that child's age.
D. *Lista de Vocabulario* [Vocabulary Checklist]	Tables 4.10–4.13; Figures 4.4–4.7	Tables 5.4–5.9	Use percentile tables for *Comprensión de Palabras* [Words Understood] and *Producción de Palabras* [Words Produced], counted separately (428 items maximum for each).
***IIª Parte: Gestos y Acciones* [Part II: Actions and Gestures]**			
Sections A through E: *Total de Gestos* [Total Gestures]	Tables 4.14 and 4.15; Figure 4.8	Tables 5.10–5.12	Use percentile tables for *Total de Gestos* [Total Gestures] (64 items), or for *Gestos Tempranos* [Early Gestures] (21 items) and *Gestos Tardíos* [Later Gestures] (43 items) computed separately.
Sections A and B: *Gestos Tempranos* [Early Gestures]	Table 4.16	Tables 5.13–5.15	
Sections C through E: *Gestos Tardíos* [Later Gestures]	Table 4.17	Tables 5.16–5.18	In most cases, *Total de Gestos* [Total Gestures] is the most appropriate, but depending on the age/level of a particular child, users may find that breakdowns into *Gestos Tempranos* [Early Gestures] and *Gestos Tardíos* [Later Gestures] provide more detailed infomation about a given child's language development.

socioeconomic status (SES) was evaluated by dividing the sample into three groups based on level of maternal education: no high school, some high school, and some college. On the basis of this classification system, 37.7% of children on Inventario I and 30.1% on Inventario II were from families whose mothers had less than a high school education. An explanation of why maternal education was chosen as an index of SES and a description of SES effects can be found in the "Maternal Education" subsection of the "Impact of Demographic Factors on Language Outcomes" section in Chapter 4. According to the 1997 Mexican Census (Instituto Nacional de Estadística, Geografía e Informática, 1997), however, 49.3% of the Mexican population has an education below junior high school level. The number of children in the Inventario norming study whose mothers have education levels below junior high school is somewhat lower (11.8% for Inventario I and 7.6% for Inventario II). *As a result, users of the Inventarios are strongly advised to use caution in applying the norms pro-*

vided in this manual to children from families in which the mother has less than a junior high school education because the norms may not be applicable.

Using the Norms with Children Who Are Learning More than One Language

Special care must be taken when using the monolingual norms with children who are learning Spanish and another language. It has been shown (Anderson, 1995; Gutierrez-Clellen, 1996; Gutiérrez-Clellen et al., 2000) that the language abilities of a bilingual child may be distributed differentially across each language. It has also been suggested that procedures formulated for using monolingual norms may not be appropriate for use with bilingual children (Anderson, 1995; Gutierrez-Clellen, 1996; Gutiérrez-Clellen et al., 2000). Pearson et al. (1995a, 1995b) and Umbel et al. (1992) have proposed that a composite score derived from both languages (discussed more later in this chapter) be used in

Table 2.4. Interpreting a child's score on Inventario II

Section of Inventario	Descriptive statistics/ developmental trends	Percentile tables	Comments/cautions
***Iª Parte: El Uso de las Palabras* [Part I: Words Children Use]**			
A. *Lista de Vocabulario* [Vocabulary Checklist]	Tables 4.17 and 4.18; Figures 4.10 and 4.11	Tables 5.19–5.21	Use percentile tables for *Producción de Palabras* [Words Produced] (690 items maximum).
B. *Cómo Usa y Comprende el Niño/a el Lenguaje* [How Children Use Words]	Tables 4.19 and 4.20; Figures 4.12 and 4.13	–	For each of 5 items, compare the response with the percentage of children with *sí* [yes] responses at the child's age.
***IIª Parte: Oraciones y Gramática* [Part II: Sentences and Grammar]**			
A. *Formas de Verbos* [*Verb Forms]	Tables 4.21 and 4.22; Figure 4.14	–	Record number of responses in each category (24 items total).
Combinación de Palabras [Combining]	Table 4.23; Figure 4.15	–	Compare response with percentage of children with a *sí* [yes] response at the child's age, with *de vez en cuando* [sometimes] or *muchas veces* [often] counted as *sí* [yes].
B. *Ejemplos* [Examples]	Table 4.24; Figures 4.16 and 4.17	Tables 5.22–5.24	Use percentile tables for *M3L-Palabras* [*M3L-Words]. Children with a *todavía no* [not yet] or a *no* [no] response to *Combinaciones* [Combining] are given an *M3L-Palabras* score of 1.0. See Table 2.2 and Appendix E for scoring procedures.
C. *Complejidad de Frases* [Complexity]	Tables 4.25 and 4.26; Figures 4.18 and 4.19	Tables 5.25–5.27	Use percentile tables for *Complejidad de Frases* [Complexity] (37 items maximum). Due to considerable range of variability in typically developing children at this age, the margin for error should be regarded as relatively wide at the months listed in the tables. Relatively small differences in percentile rankings among individual children or among groups of children should be interpreted with caution.

place of the standard scoring procedures. We agree with this proposal and have devised our scoring procedures accordingly. One advantage of having similar parent report instruments in English and Spanish, like the CDIs and Inventarios, is that composite scores can be computed, either by hand or by using the CDI Scoring Program.

A study using the CDIs and Inventarios (Marchman & Martínez-Sussmann, 2002) provided an example of the value of the composite method. In that study the vocabulary development of children living in Texas who heard both English and Spanish at least 12 hours per week ($N = 116$) was examined. Using the monolingual norms for each language, results indicated that the children had delayed language development compared with monolingual children in each language and were significantly below the 50th percentile as a group ($p < .01$) in both English and Spanish. These findings are consistent with the view that children who experience multiple language input may acquire vocabulary in each language more slowly than their monolingual peers. Following Pearson et al. (1995a, 1995b), however, a composite score was also derived based on the number of words reported on either the CDI or Inventario or both. When the composite score was used, the children demonstrated vocabulary size, as a group, that was comparable to that of monolingual peers. Further studies need to be carried out to confirm the usefulness of these instruments with a bilingual population. (See the section in Chapter 4 called "Validity of the Inventarios" for more information about the validity of the CDIs and Inventarios when used with children who are learning English and Spanish simultaneously).

Using the Norms for the Evaluation of Older Children

Many speech-language pathologists and specialists in related fields use the CDIs with children whose chronological ages exceed the upper limits of the inventories but whose language skills are within the range seen in younger typically developing children covered by the inventory norms. Recommendations for use with these populations are discussed in the subsection of Chapter 3 called "Evaluation of Older Children with Language Delay."

3

CLINICAL AND RESEARCH APPLICATIONS

CLINICAL APPLICATIONS

Many speech-language pathologists and other specialists in early intervention now use parent report to screen children for possible language delays, to help design interventions, and to track progress in speech-language therapy. Because parent report is not uniformly accurate and because it is limited to selected dimensions of development, clinical management decisions concerning an individual child should never rest solely on parent input. When the Inventarios (or any form of parent report) are used for diagnostic purposes, it is always best to "oversample" by checking the information obtained against direct observation and other types of assessment. Likewise, parent report may be used to check the findings of language samples obtained in clinical settings. Parent report often provides a more representative sample of language than is obtained in clinical settings, where spontaneous speech may be influenced by the child's shyness, the unfamiliarity of the setting, and the interaction style of the examiner. For example, many young children are reluctant to talk in the presence of unfamiliar adults. Furthermore, children rarely use all of the vocabulary words that they know in any given conversational situation. Parents are likely to have observed their children across a range of communicative situations and thus may be aware of a broader range of vocabulary and other communicative acts. Parent input is therefore an important, and even an essential, ingredient in developing a profile of an individual child's communicative skills. The Inventarios can contribute to the evaluation process as well-validated instruments that provide normed values with which a child's scores may be compared.

There are, however, some precautions regarding the use of the Inventarios for clinical purposes. These are addressed in the following sections.

Screening for Language Delay

The Inventarios have considerable potential as a preliminary screening tool for delayed language development. The usefulness of the inventories for screening the communication skills of infants and toddlers depends in large part on the age at which the child is screened and on thc manner in which the screening is conducted (i.e., static versus dynamic). Due to the enormous variability in language and communicative development in this age range, it is not possible at this time to obtain a definite diagnosis of specific language impairment during the first 3 years of life (see Leonard, 1998; Paul, 1996, 1997; and Thal & Katich, 1996, for discussions of this issue), and identification is likely to be more solid when a child is 4 than when he or she is 3 years old (Rescorla, 2000). Since the 1980s, however, research on early language delay has converged on several conventions that allow practitioners to determine whether a child is at risk for persistent language impairment. Most of the studies that have used the CDIs or other parent report instruments to study early language delay have been conducted with English-speaking children. It is not presently known whether these same models of risk for persistent language delay are valid for speakers of other languages. However, it is reasonable to use, with caution, the guidelines cited in this section when using the Inventarios to screen Spanish-speaking children until further studies on Spanish-speaking children become available.

One commonly practiced convention (known as the Delay 3 criterion, originally suggested by Rescorla, 1989) is to refer for further assessment and possible intervention any child who, according to parent report, produces fewer than 50 words or does not combine words by 24 months. Klee et al. (1998) found a disappointingly large number of overreferrals using this criterion. However, with the addition of a question about parental concerns and another about history of ear infections, Klee, Pearce, and Carson (2000) were able to significantly improve the accuracy of identification of early language delay. The practice of early identification of children with language delay is based on the finding that such children, frequently referred to as late talkers, may be at risk for language impairment (Fischel, Whitehurst, Caufield, & Debaryshe, 1989; Paul, 1996; Rescorla, 1989; Rescorla & Alley, 2001; Rescorla & Schwartz, 1990; Thal & Katich, 1996). Although there is evidence that not all late talkers will continue to have persistent language problems throughout childhood, it is recommended practice that educators and physicians refer such children for further language assessment by a certified speech-language pathologist. A screening to determine the need for further assessment is easily accomplished using Inventario II to determine whether a 24-month-old child meets the criteria proposed by Klee et al. (2000) of 1) fewer than 50 words in expressive vocabulary *or* no word combinations *and* 2) parental indication of concern about the child's language development *or* report that the child had experienced six or more ear infections during the first 2 years of life (referred to as the Delay 3+ criterion). A second convention may be employed with children younger than 2 years. This is based on the finding that delays in both production and comprehension are more predictive of risk for persistent language delays than delays in production only (Thal & Katich, 1996; Thal, Tobias, et al., 1991). This suggests that for children in this age range, production vocabulary alone is not a good predictor of later language ability and that production vocabulary scores should be interpreted in the context of comprehension vocabulary and compensatory use of gestures. That is, a child who has delays in comprehension and production and who does not make active use of gestures to assist communication is at greater risk for persistent language delay than is a child with an expressive language delay alone. These factors can be evaluated using Inventario I by comparing scores with those of typically developing children from 8 to 18 months of age.

Preliminary results (Thal, 2000) have also suggested that rates of growth in communicative behaviors during the second year of life predict later language ability better than a static assessment of these abilities at any given age. In a study of more than 1,000 children, the rate of growth in comprehension vocabulary size measured by the MacArthur CDI: Words and Gestures at three points in time from 10 to 16 months predicted children's expressive language scores at 28 months, whereas expressive or receptive vocabulary size at any one age did not. Further research that is focused on the predictive value of trajectories of development is important for validating this finding and expanding it to languages other than English.

Paul (1996) has suggested that infants and toddlers with expressive language delay should be reevaluated a number of times on a frequent basis rather than be enrolled in traditional speech-language therapy immediately after initial indentification. If the delay continues, then intensive, traditional intervention may be warranted. This recommendation is supported by the research findings reported by Thal (2000) and could be facilitated by using parent report instruments such as the CDIs or Inventarios. Both forms (Spanish and English) may be used to track a child's development of vocabulary and gesture over the course of several months while other preventive interventions, such as parent education, are employed.

Evaluation of Older Children with Language Delay

Parent report instruments, such as the CDIs, are also being used to assess the language of children whose chronological ages exceed the upper limits of the inventories but whose language skills are comparable with those of children in the age range covered by the inventories. For many applications, use of the inventories for evaluating older children with language impairments is quite appropriate (e.g., for identifying areas of strength and weaknesses for intervention and for assessing response to therapy). For example, Thal, O'Hanlon, et al. (1999) demonstrated strong validity of the English CDIs in two samples of children. In one sample, expressive vocabulary and grammar was assessed using the CDI: Words and Sentences in 39- to 49-month-old children with language delay whose scores fell below the median score for 30-month-old children. In the second, the CDI: Words and Gestures was used for assessing vocabulary production in 24- to 32-month-old children with language delays whose scores fell below the median score for 16-month-old children. Other researchers have reported the validity of the CDIs with older children with language delays of various etiologies including Down syndrome (Miller, Sedey, & Miolo, 1995), more general developmental delays (Yoder, Warren, & Biggar, 1997), and fragile X syndrome (Jackson, 1996).

The Thal, O'Hanlon, et al. (1999) findings are consonant with the suggestion by Fenson et al. (1992/1993) that the inventory scores of older children are interpretable only when the children score below the median for the oldest age group in the norming samples (18 months for Inventario I and 30 months for Inventario II). Consider the following scenario, which illustrates the limited validity with older children whose scores are above the median for the upper limit of each of the forms. Suppose the Inventario II vocabulary production score for a 42-month-old boy was 353 words. The most appropriate reference level is always the median or 50th percentile level. As shown in Table 5.21 in Chapter 5, it would be appropriate to say that the child's productive vocabulary is equivalent to that of a 28-month-old boy with typically developing language. In a sense, we are justified in saying that the 42-month-old child has a "language age" equivalent to the 28-month level. Suppose, however, that the same 42-month-old boy is reported to produce 660 words (i.e., near the Inventario II ceiling). It would not be appropriate to conclude that this child's language is equivalent to that of a precocious 30-month-old, nor would it be appropriate to conclude that the child is doing well. Other researchers (e.g., Bishop, 1997; Lahey, 1988; Lawrence, 1992) have pointed out the psychometric limitations of age-equivalence scores for comparing children's scores with those of test norms. In short, use of the inventories with children older than 30 months who have developmental delays is recommended only when the scores do not exceed the median 30-month scores on Inventario II (or the median 18-month scores when Inventario I is used). Literal interpretation of scores for any children must be done with caution. For children with scores above the 30-month median, other tests should be used because interpretation of the inventory scores could result in serious underestimation of communicative skills as a result of ceiling effects.

Although the convention of estimating an approximate language age for older children whose scores fall below the norming sample median for 30-month-old children for CDI: Words and Sentences (or for 18-month-old children for CDI: Words and Gestures) was devised for the English CDIs, this procedure could also be applied to the Inventarios with Spanish-speaking children. As with the English CDIs, however, caution should be exercised in characterizing the language level of an older child to avoid under- and overestimations of the child's communicative skills.

Formulation of Intervention Strategies

The development of a communicative profile for a child through the use of the Inventarios can also contribute to the identification of aspects of the child's communicative skills that may be targeted for intervention. These may include broad domains such as vocabulary production or specific ones such as particular semantic or syntactic categories. One precaution should be taken in using the Inventarios for this purpose. In a study of English-speaking children with developmental delays, Yoder et al. (1997) found that the test–retest reliability of the CDI across a 2-week interval was excellent for the total number of words understood but inadequate for individual items. The degree to which mothers were inconsistent in reporting particular vocabulary items varied as a function of the types of words they were reporting. For example, mothers' reports of words *understood* tended to be more stable for nouns than for descriptive words. This suggests that the Inventarios are best used to identify overall vocabulary delays but not to identify specific words for remediation. The case may be different, however, with respect to *production* of specific words. Clinicians may wish to use the Inventarios to identify classes of words that appear to require remediation and supplement these findings with more targeted behavioral assessments of individual words.

Evaluation of Intervention Effects

Because parent report is based on a variety of contexts outside the clinic or laboratory, it can be useful for monitoring changes as a result of intervention. In order to demonstrate that therapy has been effective, evidence concerning performance outside of the intervention context is essential. Parents are uniquely positioned to provide this important information. The CDIs have been used in clinical intervention studies to track the effects of intervention on English-speaking children with expressive language delay (Girolametto, Pearce, & Weitzman, 1996, 1997; Girolametto, Weitzman, Wiigs, & Pearce, 1999; Robertson & Weismer, 1999) or cleft lip and/or palate (Scherer, 1999) and to examine the effects of cochlear implant use in a child with hearing loss (Willis & Edwards, 1996). The Inventarios are expected to serve the same purpose for Spanish-speaking children.

RESEARCH APPLICATIONS

The ease with which the Inventarios can be administered makes possible a global assessment of language for larger samples of children than previously has been possible. Below are some research applications that follow from this capability.

Screening and Preselection of Children at Different Levels of Language Development

Researchers are often interested in studying children who are at a specific point in the language acquisition process or in tracking them from the onset of a specified milestone. A researcher interested in following the passage from first words to grammar can start with a group of children defined by age and use one of the Inventarios to determine which children meet the desired "starting point" criterion in language development (e.g., producing fewer than 50 words).

Screening and Preselection of Children with Particular Language Characteristics or Children with Unusual Profiles

The Inventarios permit identification of late talkers (e.g., Klee et al., 1998; Klee et al., 2000; Rescorla, 1989; Thal & Bates, 1988), early talkers (e.g., Dale, Bates, Reznick, & Morisset, 1989; Thal, Bates, Zappia, & Oroz, 1996), and children with other specific profiles. The Inventarios may also be used to select children with unusual configurations of linguistic and nonlinguistic abilities (e.g., children whose comprehension far exceeds their production; Bates, Thal, Whitesell, Fenson, & Oakes, 1989; Benedict, 1979; Snyder, Bates, & Bretherton, 1981), children who are reported to gesture extensively despite language delays, and children who are surprisingly slow to produce word combinations despite their vocabulary level.

Matching Children on Language Skills

In many instances, it is important for researchers to ensure that groups are initially equivalent in communicative skills, such as when investigating the effects of specific environmental factors or intervention experiences in pre- and posttest designs. The Inventarios provide researchers with an efficient means for matching children on the basis of vocabulary size and/or utterance length.

Examination of the Influence of Other Variables on Language Development

The Inventarios permit the collection of data from relatively large samples to assess the effects on language of such global variables as family size, socioeconomic status, ethnicity, birth order, child-rearing practices, type of day-today care used, and number of languages spoken in the home. Such studies have been carried out using the CDIs with English-speaking children from a variety of backgrounds (e.g., Arriaga, Fenson, Cronan, & Pethick, 1998; Bornstein & Haynes, 1998; Bornstein et al., 1998; Feldman et al., 2000; Huebner, 2000; Roberts, Burchinal, & Durham, 1999; Saxon, 1997). Similarly, Laakso, Poikkeus, Eklund, and Lyytinen (1999) and Lyytinen, Poikkeus, Leiwo, Ahonen, and Lyytinen (1996) have used a Finnish version of the CDIs to examine parenting styles on the language development of Finnish-speaking children.

4

TECHNICAL INFORMATION

PHASES OF DEVELOPMENT OF THE INVENTARIOS

Origins of the Instruments

The Inventarios have been developed over a period of more than 25 years and can be traced back to research by Bates and her colleagues in Rome during the early 1970s (Bates et al., 1975). By the late 1980s, the English instruments had evolved into a set of four forms, each designed to cover a relatively narrow age range. Those instruments were the Communicative Development Questionnaire (8–12 months), the Language and Gesture Inventory (12–18 months), the Early Language Inventory (18–27 months), and the Grammatical Development Questionnaire (24–36 months). These versions evolved into the MacArthur Communicative Development Inventories (CDIs), a pair of instruments for English-speaking children with reliable and valid norms that are widely used for clinical and research purposes (Dale, 1991, 1996; Dale et al., 1989; Fenson et al., 1992/1993). The Italian versions were developed in parallel with the English ones and were formally published a short time later (Caselli & Casadio, 1995). The CDIs have also been adapted to and normed in many other languages (see the page about adaptations on the CDI web site, http://www.sci.sdsu.edu/cdi/foreign.html, for a current list and authors).

Early Development of the Inventarios

The Spanish forms were adapted linguistically and culturally from the English and Italian versions of the MacArthur inventories. New words were added to the *Lista de Vocabulario* [Vocabulary Checklist], and sections were modified to reflect cross-linguistic differences in grammatical categories. For example, Inventario II has a separate section, *Estados* [*State Verbs], about the three state verbs, *ser, estar,* and *haber,* whereas the English CDI: Words and Sentences has a separate section called Helping Verbs. In addition, the categories into which prepositions, locatives, quantifiers, articles, and adverbs are organized differ across the languages. The second part of Inventario II, *Oraciones y Gramática* [Sentences and Grammar], was completely revised to reflect properties that are specific to the Spanish language.

The *Lista de Vocabulario* [Vocabulary Checklist] for both Inventario I and II was based primarily on naturalistic language data from a series of Spanish acquisition studies conducted in the United States and Mexico (Eisenberg, 1985; González, 1983; Gutiérrez, 1976; Jackson, 1989) and from experiments carried out at the University of the Americas in Mexico City (Jackson-Maldonado, unpublished data). The English and Italian checklists, as well as standardized tests such as the Test de Vocabulario en Imágenes Peabody, Adaptación Hispano-americana (Dunn et al., 1986); the Batería de Evaluación Intelectual Kaufman (Kaufman, Kaufman, Gómez Palacio, Rangel, & Padilla, 1987); the WISC-RM: Wechsler Intelligence Scale for Children–Revised (Mexicano; Gómez Palacio, Padilla, & Roll, 1982); and the Batería de Evaluación de la Lengua Española (Gómez Palacio, 1988) were examined to identify additional words that were culturally, developmentally, and linguistically appropriate.

All items were screened for linguistic and cultural relevance to ensure appropriateness for Mexican and Mexican American populations. Cultural modifications included the addition of Mexican games and routines, such as *ojitos* and *tortillitas;* Mexican foods, such as *chile* and *tortilla* (and items for Hispanics in the United States, e.g., *peanut butter*); and people such as *madrina,* and the omission of words such as *basement, backyard,* and *sandbox.* Because Spanish is a morphologically rich language, several categories of items were expanded to reflect gender and number in articles and pronouns, and gender in adjectives. For instance, the Spanish definite article has four forms (*el, la, los, las*), whereas there is only one definite article in English (*the*).

Preliminary versions (Jackson-Maldonado et al., 1993) of the Inventarios contained a vocabulary and gesture use checklist and several grammatical scales. Forms were completed by parents of 328 healthy children ($n = 138$ for Inventario I from 8 to 16 months of age, and $n = 190$ for Inventario II from 15 to 31 months of age) who resided primarily in the southwestern part of the United States.

Language sample data for 17 participants were collected to assess the validity of these instruments. Results indicated a strong correlation ($r = .84, p < .0001$) between *Producción de Palabras* [Words Produced] on Inventario II and the number of different words produced in a language sample. Test–retest reliability was assessed by comparing inventories completed by 16 mothers at an interval of 1 month. These data also provided evidence of reliability ($r = .62$ for word production) similar to results obtained with the English CDI. It was also found that vocabulary growth and lexical composition as measured by the Spanish Inventarios were very similar to those found for English using the English instruments. For a full description of these and other results, see Jackson-Maldonado et al. (1993).

Development of the Present Instruments

The preliminary norms just described provided sufficient evidence of validity and reliability to motivate a larger norming study. Several modifications were made to the instruments to produce the final versions. First, because many parents had not completed the grammatical scales on the preliminary forms, steps were taken to make this section more user-friendly. Second, we eliminated items on the *Lista de Vocabulario* [Vocabulary Checklist] that had not been checked by any of the parents. Third, we included similar numbers of words per section on the *Lista de Vocabulario* [Vocabulary Checklist] as are found in versions in other languages (when doing so was reasonable) so that cross-linguistic comparisons would be more reliable. Finally, we developed a grammar complexity section that was designed to be appropriate for Spanish and comparable to CDIs in other languages. The new forms, Inventario del Desarrollo de Habilidades Comunicativas: Primeras Palabras y Gestos (Inventario I) and Inventario del Desarrollo de Habilidades Comunicativas: Palabras y Enunciados (Inventario II), were then administered to a sample of more than 2,000 children; the data from this sample form the basis for the norms provided in this manual.

THE NORMING STUDY

Data Collection

Data for the norming study were collected by trained research assistants (RAs) who were students in psychology, linguistics, or communication disorders. The method of data collection was determined by the educational level of the children's mothers following one of three procedures.

1. For a mother with some schooling (at any level) who was willing and able to fill out the forms on her own (approximately 80% of the sample)
    a. Brief instructions and examples of what was meant by comprehension were given.
    b. Different examples of what was meant by production were provided.
    c. The Inventario was then given to the mother to complete.
    d. The form was collected at a later date, no longer than 2 weeks after the day it was given to the mother. No forms were returned by mail. All were picked up by an RA either from the parent directly or from a child care center or clinic.
2. For a mother who was illiterate or who had a low level of education and was uncomfortable filling out the forms (approximately 5% of the participants)
    a. The Inventario was completed with the help of an RA.
    b. If the mother was also reluctant to fill out the forms, the RA did so following the mother's oral response to each item.
    c. In exceptional cases, the form was explained to another member of the family, who filled out the form with the mother.

3. For a mother whose child attended a child care center and who could not be contacted directly (approximately 15% of the participants)
    a. Instructions for completing the form were given to the child care teachers, who distributed the form to the mother. (Although the teachers were asked to provide appropriate instruction to each mother, some teachers reported that they did not consistently do so.)
    b. These forms were collected during a later visit to the center.

Sampling Procedure

Children were recruited through friends, neighbors, family members, acquaintances, staff at private child care centers, staff at public child care centers (the Instituto Mexicano del Seguro Social and the Department of Desarrollo Integral de la Familia), pediatricians, community clinic staff, social workers in villages, clergy, hospital waiting room staff, and on the street or in parks. Some participants were part of research projects addressing other issues at the Universidad Autónoma de Querétaro, the Universidad Autónoma de San Luís Potosí, and the University of the Americas in Mexico City. The total population for the norming study resided in the cities of Aguascalientes, Celaya (Guanajuato), Guanajuato, Los Mochis (Sinaloa), Mexico City, Querétaro, San Luís Potosí, and San Miguel Allende (Guanajuato). Our goal was to obtain a sample with a minimum of 60 children for each of the 26 age groups (i.e., at least 660 children for Inventario I and 900 children for Inventario II) and a minimum of 30 girls and 30 boys for each age group, from a variety of socioeconomic levels.

Table 4.1. Number of children by age and sex in the norming sample: Inventario I

Age in months	Sex	
	Girls (*n*)	Boys (*n*)
8	34	37
9	28	31
10	35	42
11	32	33
12	46	50
13	40	40
14	42	33
15	30	36
16	31	29
17	30	37
18	25	37
Total	**373**	**405**

Table 4.2. Number of children by age and sex in the norming sample: Inventario II

Age in months	Sex	
	Girls (*n*)	Boys (*n*)
16	35	34
17	31	27
18	31	31
19	37	34
20	45	48
21	38	46
22	26	31
23	47	41
24	40	35
25	29	41
26	32	41
27	38	34
28	39	43
29	44	31
30	29	36
Total	**541**	**553**

Table 4.3. Education level of mothers in the norming sample compared with educational level for the Mexican population (ages 15 and older)

Education level	Mexican population (%)[a]	Inventario I (%)	Inventario II (%)
No schooling	10.4	2.0	0.7
Primary school	38.9	9.8	6.9
Junior high school	21.8	23.2	22.5
High school	17.2	31.7	31.0
College/university	11.0	33.4	39.0

[a]Mexican demographic information was obtained from the 1997 Mexican census (Instituto Nacional de Estadística, Geografía e Informática,1997).

Medical Exclusion Criteria

Data were collected from a total of 818 children between 8 and 18 months of age for Inventario I and 1,125 children between 16 and 30 months of age for Inventario II. Subsequently, 40 children were excluded from the Inventario I sample and 31 children were excluded from the Inventario II sample for medical reasons, including low birth weight (less than 2,300 grams) and serious hospitalizations or medical conditions. The final sample size consisted of 778 children between 8 and 18 months of age for Inventario I (see Table 4.1) and 1,094 children between 16 and 30 months of age for Inventario II (see Table 4.2).

Demographic Distribution of the Sample

On the basis of information reported by the participating families, participants in the norming samples for Inventarios I and II were evaluated in terms of maternal education, birth order, and exposure to a second language.

Maternal Education Table 4.3 shows mothers' level of education for both samples (Inventario I and Inventario II) compared with the education level of all people ages 15 and older living in Mexico (Instituto Nacional de Estadísitica, Geografía e Informática, 1997). Both samples show an upward educational bias relative to national demographics. This bias was even more pronounced in the norming sample for the English CDIs (see Table 4-3 on p. 43 of Fenson et al., 1992/1993), in which more than 77% of the population had some college education. This led the authors of the CDIs to conclude that the English norms were likely to be representative of children whose mothers have at least a high school education but that the norms may not be applicable to children from families with low levels of education and income. These cautions are appropriate for the current sample as well. At the same time, Table 4.4 shows that the Spanish sample is evenly distributed across the three education categories in the norming sample analyses (i.e., no high school, some high school, some college), with about one third of the sample representing parents with no high school or college experience. See the subsection later in this chapter called "Maternal Education" for discussion of the impact of these factors on specific language milestones assessed by the Inventarios.

Table 4.4. Demographic profile comparison of the English MacArthur Communicative Development Inventory (CDI) and the Spanish Inventario norming samples

Maternal education	English CDIs (%)[a]	Spanish Inventarios (%)
No high school	0	32.1
Some high school	22.4	31.3
Some college	77.6	36.6

[a]*Source:* Table 4-3 on page 43 of Fenson et al. (1992/1993). Some percentages are combined in this table to allow comparison with the Spanish Inventario samples.

Birth Order Table 4.5 shows the percentage of children by reported birth order for the Inventario I and Inventario II norming samples. The majority of children were either first- or second-born, with approximately one fifth of the children in both samples being later-born. For more information about the impact of birth order on the major language skills assessed by the Inventarios, see the subsection later in this chapter called "Birth Order."

Table 4.5. Birth order of the children in the norming sample

Birth order	Inventario I (%)	Inventario II (%)
First-born	44.3	48.0
Second-born	33.0	31.7
Later-born	22.7	20.3

Exposure to a Second Language The norming study was limited to children for whom Mexican Spanish was the primary language. Forms were accepted, however, for children who were exposed to more than one language. In the Inventario I sample, 6.2% of the children were reported to be exposed to a second language. Exposure to a second language was reported for 10.1% of the Inventario II sample. Overall, 8.9% of the total sample (both Inventarios combined) had exposure to more than one language. This level is comparable to that reported for the English norming sample, in which 12.2% of the children were reported to have some exposure to a second language.

DEVELOPMENTAL TRENDS IN COMMUNICATIVE DEVELOPMENT

This section provides an overview of the growth of the major features of communicative development across the 8- to 30-month age range represented by the two Spanish inventories (Inventario I and Inventario II). On the basis of data from the norming of the Inventarios, developmental trends are presented, including the growth of vocabulary, use of gestures, and the emergence and expansion of grammar.

Statistical Methods

The developmental trends were examined using the following statistical methods.

Descriptive Statistics Descriptive statistics for each section of the inventories at each month of age are displayed in Tables 4.7–4.26. The descriptive statistics include the number of children, mean, median, standard deviation, and minimum and maximum scores observed at each month. A graphic representation of the mean scores of each variable by month is also provided for many sections of each of the Inventarios. In such figures, the bars above and below each mean score represent the 95.5% confidence intervals. The text accompanying the tables and graphs gives brief descriptions of the vocabulary skills highlighted by the descriptive statistics. In addition, some of the tables show the percentage of children who obtained scores within successive ranges (e.g., 0–100, 101–200), providing further information on the variability in communicative skills for the 8- to 30-month age span. (*Note:* In some cases, percentages do not add up to 100.0 due to rounding.)

Inferential Statistics Analyses of variance were carried out to determine the effects of age and sex and their possible interaction for several key variables. On Inventario I, measures include *Comprensión de las Primeras Frases* [Phrases Understood], *Comprensión de Palabras* [Words Understood], *Producción de Palabras* [Words Produced], and *Total de Gestos* [Total Gestures]. On Inventario II, analyses involve *Producción de Palabras* [Words Produced], *M3L-Palabras* [M3L-*Words], and *Complejidad de Frases* [Complexity]. Partial eta squared (η^2) was used to determine the magnitude of each effect in terms of variance accounted for by each significant factor. Modified Bonferroni corrections (Keppel, 1991) were applied in tests of the differences between boys and girls at each month for each of these seven measures. The alpha level was set at $p < .005$ for Inventario I and at $p < .003$ for Inventario II to control for the Type I family-wise error rate in each of the simple effect t-tests performed.

Curve Fitting Growth-curve modeling was used to capture the pattern of the increase in language skills over age. This technique uses all of the data simultaneously to show overall patterns of development and to predict scores (Burchinal & Appelbaum, 1991). Growth-curve fitting is similar to the technique of linear regression but without the restriction that the end result must be a straight line. Instead, growth-curve modeling is an extension of linear regression, encompassing a wider range of mathematical functions than just straight lines, and is often used for models of growth (Fenson et al., 1994). The logistic function was used for most of the data described here because logistic functions typically begin with a gradual increment, leading to a more rapid surge, followed by a leveling off, a pattern typically observed in the acquisition of language and in other developmental domains (Burchinal & Appelbaum, 1991).

Percentile Scores Percentile scores in increments of 5, starting with the 5th percentile and ending at the 99th percentile, were calculated for both sexes combined and for boys and girls separately. Using these percentile scores, fitted scores were calculated using the logistic growth-curve function. The fitted percentile scores for *Comprensión de las Primeras Frases* [Phrases Understood], *Comprensión de Palabras* [Words Understood], *Producción de Palabras* [Words Produced], *Total de Gestos* [Total Gestures], *Gestos Tempranos* [Early Ges-

Table 4.6. Percentage of children with zero to one, two, or three *sí* [yes] responses on *Comprensión Temprana* [First Signs of Understanding] (Inventario I)

Age in months	Girls: Number of *sí* [yes] responses			Boys: Number of *sí* [yes] responses		
	0–1	2	3	0–1	2	3
8	8.8	20.6	70.6	2.7	21.6	75.7
9	3.6	7.1	89.3	3.2	12.9	83.9
10	2.9	0	97.1	2.4	26.2	71.4
11	0	3.1	96.9	12.2	6.1	81.8
12	4.4	13.0	82.6	4.0	10.0	86.0
13	0	5.0	95.0	0	12.5	87.5
14	0	14.3	85.7	6.0	12.1	81.8
15	0	10.0	90.0	2.8	2.8	94.4
16	0	9.7	90.3	3.4	10.3	86.2
17	0	10.0	90.0	0	10.8	89.2
18	0	4.0	96.0	0	5.4	94.6

tures], and *Gestos Tardíos* [Later Gestures] on Inventario I and for *Producción de Palabras* [Words Produced], *Complejidad de Frases* [Complexity], and *M3L-Palabras* [M3L-*Words] on Inventario II are shown in tabular form in Chapter 5. The growth curves for the 90th, 75th, 50th, 25th, and 10th percentiles are also depicted graphically in Chapter 5.

Inventario I Components

Developmental trends in communicative development for each of the components of Inventario I are presented in this part of the manual. Each section of Inventario I is presented with the Spanish name as it appears on the Inventario and on the *Informe del Niño/a* [Child Report Form]. As mentioned in Chapter 1, English glosses are provided in square brackets; an asterisk marks a section that does not have a counterpart on the CDI: Words and Gestures.

***Comprensión Temprana* [First Signs of Understanding]** *Comprensión Temprana* [First Signs of Understanding] was designed to assess rudimentary signs of understanding in infants who may not yet show evidence of specific word comprehension. Table 4.6 presents the proportion of children at each age who were reported to have zero to one, two, or three *sí* [yes] responses. The results indicate that more than 70% of children were reported to be exhibiting each of these three behaviors by 8 months of age. The proportion of children with three "behavior present" responses increased to more than 80% at 10 months and 90% at 11 months. These early signs of language comprehension were clearly typical of the vast majority of children across the age range sampled here. Similarly high levels were observed in the norming sample of the English CDI. Although this measure may not serve to clearly discriminate among the children in this sample, parents may nevertheless appreciate this opportunity to comment on their child's burgeoning communicative skills. Furthermore, children who do not show these early signs of understanding may be at risk for later language and/or cognitive delays.

***Comprensión de las Primeras Frases* [Phrases Understood]** Figure 4.1 shows the mean *Comprensión de las Primeras Frases* [Phrases Understood] scores reported for children from 8 to 18 months of age. The growth curve is monotonic (i.e., they increase regularly across the relevant age range) except for a slight dip at 17 months. The confidence intervals indicate relatively constant variation throughout the age period.

More complete descriptive statistics for *Comprensión de las Primeras Frases* [Phrases Understood] are presented in Table 4.7. As was the case with the analogous section on the English CDI (see Table 4-6 on p. 49 of Fenson et al., 1992/1993), understanding of phrases was reported on Inventario I as early as 8 or 9 months of age, with a steady increase in the number of items reported across the Inventario I age range. Also note, however, that the standard deviations are fairly substantial at each monthly interval for this measure, indicating that there is considerable variation within the sample of children at each age.

Table 4.8 further highlights the variation in the number of phrases that were reported to be comprehended by 8- to 18-month-old Spanish-speaking children. Here, we present the proportion of children with 0, 1–10, 11–20, and 21–28 phrases understood at each monthly interval. At virtually all ages, some children were reported to understand very few phrases, whereas other children approached or reached the ceiling level of 28 phrases. By 10 months, however, more than half of the children were reported to produce 11–20 of the phrases

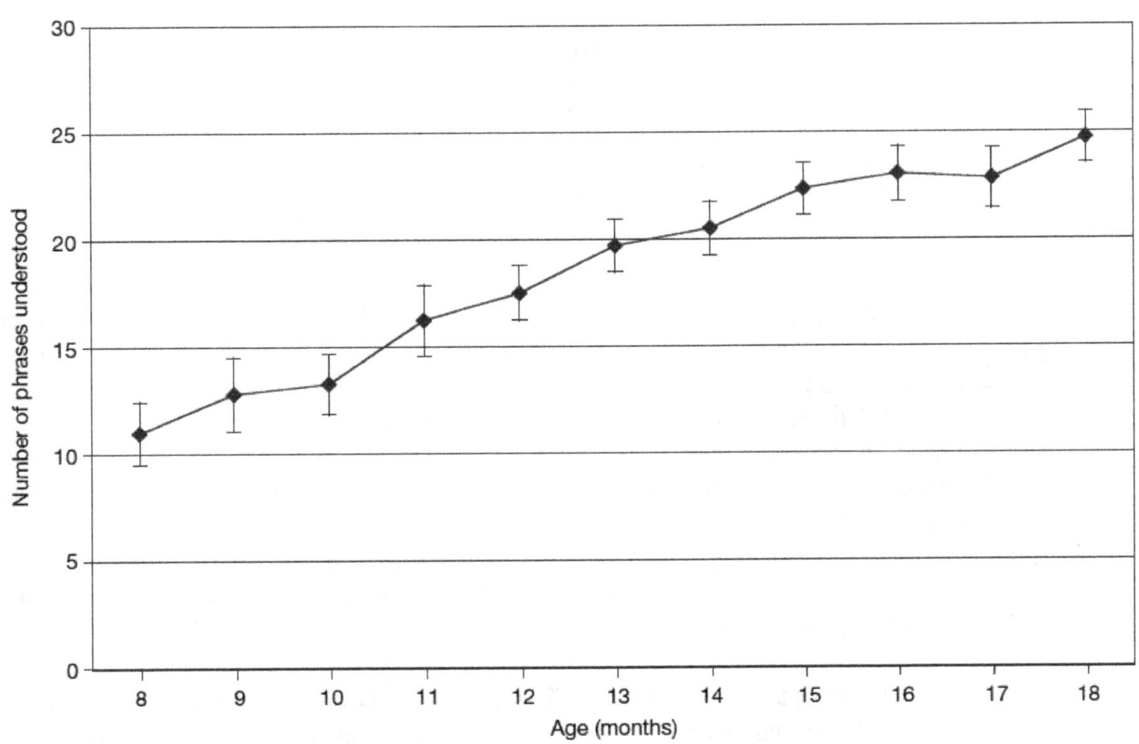

Figure 4.1. Mean *Comprensión de las Primeras Frases* [Phrases Understood] (Inventario I) scores by age in months. (*Note:* Bars above and below each mean score represent the 95.5% confidence intervals.)

Table 4.7. Descriptive statistics for *Comprensión de las Primeras Frases* [Phrases Understood] (Inventario I)

Age in months	*n*	Mean	Median	Standard deviation	Minimum	Maximum[a]
8	71	11.0	11.0	6.2	1	26
9	59	12.8	13.0	6.6	2	26
10	77	13.3	13.0	6.2	0	27
11	65	16.3	17.0	6.7	3	28
12	96	17.5	18.0	6.3	3	28
13	80	19.7	20.0	5.5	7	28
14	75	20.5	20.0	5.5	3	28
15	66	22.4	23.0	4.9	8	28
16	60	23.1	24.0	5.0	11	28
17	67	22.8	25.0	5.8	4	28
18	62	24.7	27.0	4.7	3	28

[a]Maximum score possible = 28.

Table 4.8. Percentage of children with *Comprensión de las Primeras Frases* [Phrases Understood] (Inventario I) scores falling in four successive ranges

Age in months	*Comprensión de las Primeras Frases* [Phrases Understood] scores[a]			
	0	1–10	11–20	21–28
8	0	46.5	43.7	9.9
9	0	39.0	45.8	15.3
10	1.3	28.6	58.4	11.7
11	0	23.1	52.3	24.6
12	0	13.5	53.1	33.3
13	0	5.0	48.8	46.3
14	0	4.0	46.7	49.3
15	0	1.5	25.8	72.7
16	0	0	28.3	71.7
17	0	4.5	23.9	71.6
18	0	1.6	12.9	85.5

[a]Maximum score possible = 28.

listed. By 14 months, almost half (49%) of the children understood 21–28 of the phrases. By 18 months, almost all of the children in the sample (86%) understood the majority of the phrases (i.e., 21–28 phrases).

Figure 4.2 depicts the mean *Comprensión de las Primeras Frases* [Phrases Understood] scores separately for boys and girls at each month. A 2 (sex) × 11 (age) between-subjects analysis of variance on number of phrases understood yielded a significant main effect for age $F(10, 756) = 43.54$, $p < .01$, no significant main effect of sex, $F(1, 756) = 2.87$, *ns*, and no significant interaction, $F(10, 756) = 1.698$, *ns*. Age accounted for 35% of the variance. The percentiles by age and gender for this measure are presented in Tables 5.1–5.3 in Chapter 5.

***Maneras de Hablar* [Starting to Talk]** This section asks how often a child imitates words or parts of sentences and how often a child names or labels objects. Responses of *de vez en cuando* [sometimes] and *muchas veces* [often] were combined as *sí* [yes], to be contrasted with *todavía no* [not yet] responses.

The percentage of children at each month with *sí* [yes] responses for *Imita* [Imitation] and *Nombra* [Labeling] is shown in Table 4.9 and Figure 4.3. Imitation was more common than labeling at each monthly level. Both behaviors showed an increasing developmental trend, although growth in the number of children reported to label objects did not begin until after 11 months. No significant differences were observed in the frequency of imitating or labeling between boys and girls at any month.

Table 4.9. Percentage of children with *sí* [yes] responses for *Imita* [Imitation] and *Nombra* [Labeling] in *Maneras de Hablar* [First Signs of Talking] (Inventario I)

	Maneras de Hablar [First Signs of Talking]	
Age in months	*Imita* [Imitation]	*Nombra* [Labeling]
8	31.0	15.5
9	42.4	18.6
10	50.6	20.8
11	50.8	16.9
12	63.5	38.5
13	71.3	52.5
14	60.0	44.0
15	74.2	56.1
16	78.3	65.0
17	79.1	70.1
18	83.9	75.8

***Lista de Vocabulario* [Vocabulary Checklist]** Based on the responses in the *Lista de Vocabulario* [Vocabulary Checklist], Figure 4.4 presents *Comprensión de Palabras* [Words Understood] reported as the mean number of words understood by age in months. This figure shows a gradual, monotonically increasing trend in the number of reported words understood from 9 months through 17 months, leveling off at this point. The confidence intervals indicate

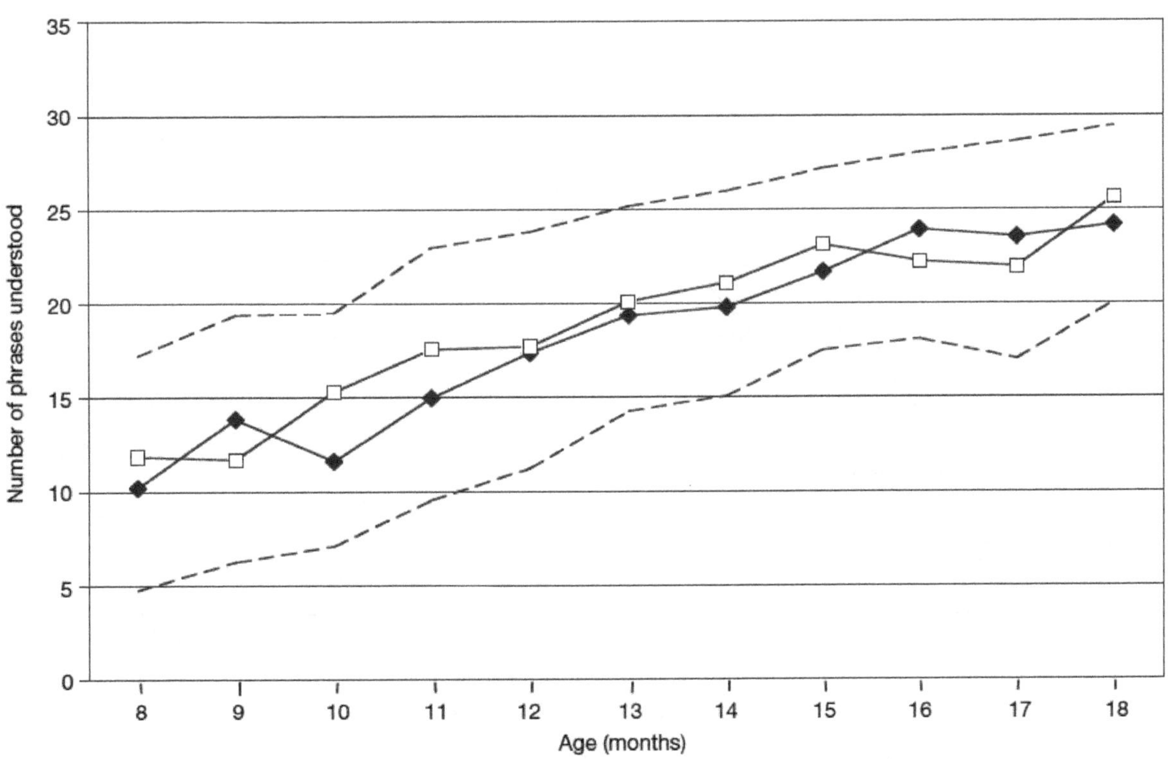

Figure 4.2. Mean *Comprensión de las Primeras Frases* [Phrases Understood] (Inventario I) scores by age and sex. (*Note:* The dashed line represents ±1 standard deviation for the sexes combined.) (*Key:* —◆— boys; —□— girls.)

fairly consistent variability across age, although there was some tendency for the variation to be somewhat larger in the later months. We can note that the level of vocabulary comprehension observed in the present sample of Spanish-speaking children is generally comparable to that reported for English-speaking infants (see Figure 4-3 on p. 48 of Fenson et al., 1992/1993).

Table 4.10 presents more complete descriptive statistics for *Comprensión de Palabras* [Words Understood] by age in months. Mean scores exceeded 50 words at the 3 earliest months and increased steadily thereafter to a mean of more than 200 words at 17 and 18 months. For the first 7 monthly levels (8–14 months), at least one child was reported to not understand any words. No child reached the ceiling of 428 words until 16 months. There is considerable variation in vocabulary comprehension levels across the age range, especially in the later months. The fitted percentile scores for this measure can be found in Tables 5.4–5.6 in Chapter 5.

Variability among Spanish-speaking children in *Comprensión de Palabras* [Words Understood] can be further seen in Table 4.11. This table presents the percentage of children at each age with reported comprehension scores falling in five successive vocabulary ranges: 0–100, 101–200, 201–300, 301–400, and 401–428 words. Note that most children in the sample fell in the middle ranges of possible scores at all ages, with only a few children reaching the highest levels at the older ages.

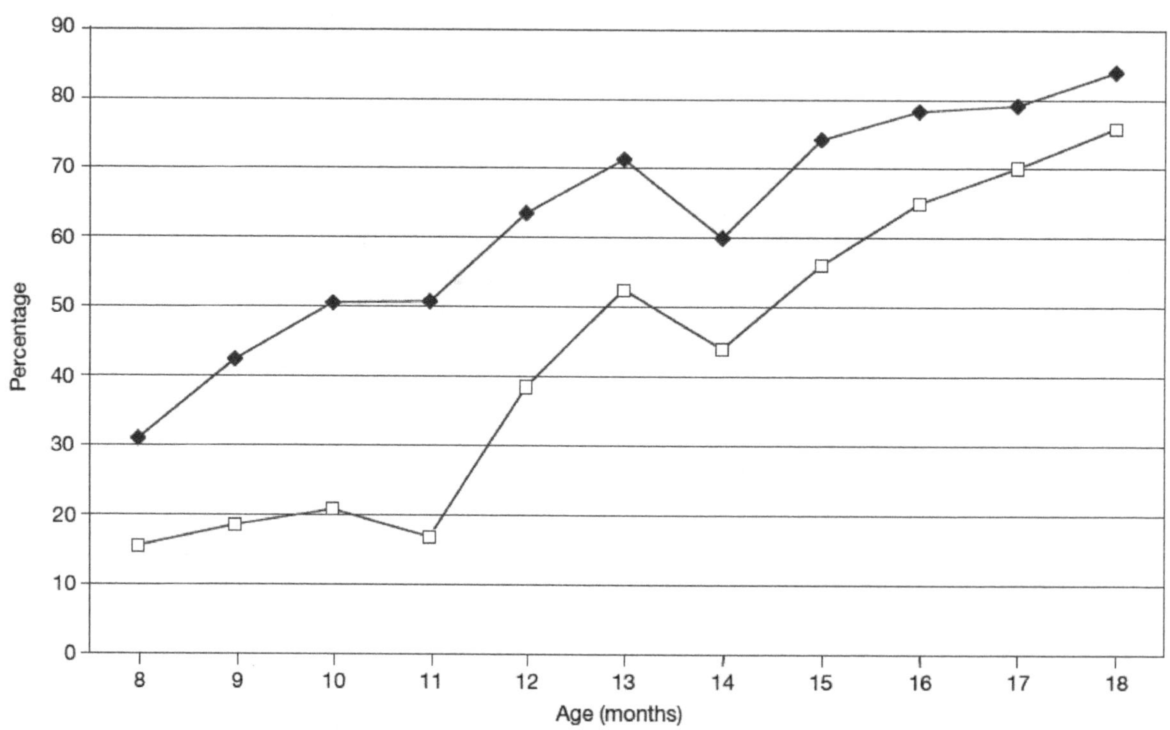

Figure 4.3. Percentage of children with *sí* [yes] responses for *Imita* [Imitation] and *Nombra* [Labeling] in *Maneras de Hablar* [Starting to Talk] (Inventario I) by age in months. (*Key:* —◆— Imitation; —□— Labeling.)

Comprensión de Palabras [Words Understood] for boys and girls at each age is shown in Figure 4.5 as mean number of words understood. These scores were evaluated with a 2 (sex) × 11 (age) between-subjects analysis of variance. There was a significant main effect of age, $F(10, 756) = 33.5, p < .001$. The main effect of sex, however, was not significant, $F(1, 756) = .70$, *ns*, nor was the interaction between sex and age, $F(10, 756) = .84$, *ns*. Age accounted for 30% of the variance.

Turning to *Producción de Palabras* [Words Produced], Figure 4.6 presents the mean number of reported words produced (for both sexes combined) by age in months. This figure shows a gradual, monotonically increasing trend from 8 to 18 months. The mean score for vocabulary production did not exceed 20 words until 14 months, yet by 18 months, the average child was reported to produce approximately 58 words. The confidence intervals suggest relatively narrow ranges of scores early on but quite substantial variation in the later months. The growth trend for Spanish-speaking infants is generally comparable to that reported by Fenson et al. (1992/1993) for English-speaking infants up to about 13 months. Beyond this point, the mean number of words produced is higher for the children from the English CDI sample (see Figure 4-4 on p. 49 in Fenson et al., 1992/1993). This may be a reflection of the generally higher socioeconomic level of the infants in the norming sample for the English CDI. (See the comparison of English and Spanish samples based on mother's level of education in Table 4.4 and the discussion of the relationship between educational

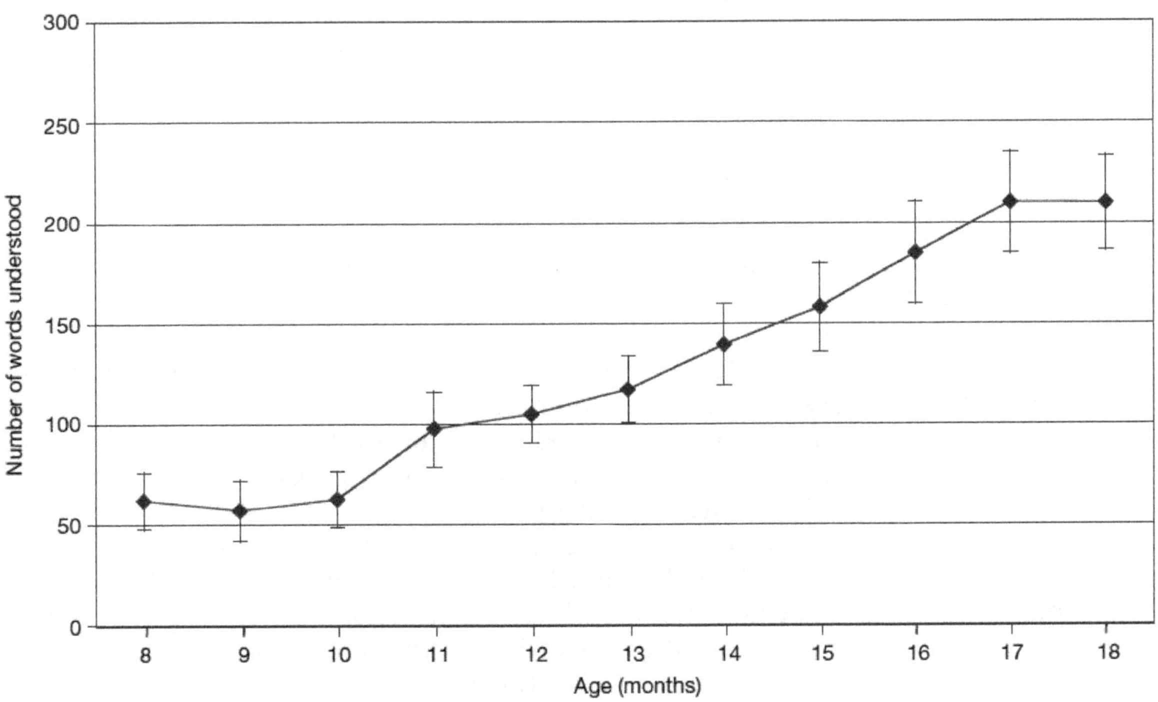

Figure 4.4. Mean *Comprensión de Palabras* [Words Understood] (Inventario I) scores by age in months. (*Note:* Bars above and below each mean score represent the 95.5% confidence intervals.)

Table 4.10. Descriptive statistics for *Comprensión de Palabras* [Words Understood] (Inventario I)

Age in months	*n*	Mean	Median	Standard deviation	Minimum	Maximum[a]
8	71	62.0	43.0	59.6	0	241
9	59	57.1	34.0	58.4	0	224
10	77	62.7	43.0	60.6	0	349
11	65	97.6	85.0	75.3	0	292
12	96	104.8	87.0	69.7	0	280
13	80	117.1	111.0	74.3	0	334
14	75	139.4	142.0	87.2	0	374
15	66	157.8	141.5	89.5	17	417
16	60	185.1	182.5	98.2	19	428
17	67	210.0	210.0	103.6	6	424
18	62	209.7	207.0	91.9	28	424

[a]Maximum score possible = 428.

Table 4.11. Percentage of children with *Comprensión de Palabras* [Words Understood] (Inventario I) scores falling in five successive ranges

Age in months	*Comprensión de Palabras* [Words Understood][a]				
	0–100	101–200	201–300	301–400	401–428
8	77.5	18.3	4.2	0	0
9	81.4	16.9	1.7	0	0
10	76.6	20.8	1.3	1.3	0
11	61.5	24.6	13.8	0	0
12	54.2	35.4	10.4	0	0
13	46.3	40.0	12.5	1.3	0
14	36.0	44.0	17.3	2.7	0
15	30.3	39.4	25.8	3.0	1.5
16	20.0	45.0	20.0	11.7	3.3
17	14.9	31.3	31.3	16.4	6.0
18	9.7	37.1	37.1	12.9	3.2

[a]Maximum score possible = 428.

level and vocabulary outcome in the subsection later in this chapter called "Maternal Education.")

Complete descriptive statistics for *Producción de Palabras* [Words Produced] are presented in Table 4.12. At all months, the standard deviations are larger than their respective means, highlighting the wide variability in the distribution of scores for vocabulary production across the age range. This phenomenon is also seen in the English CDI sample (see Figure 4-4 on p. 49 of Fenson et al., 1992/1993). Percentile tables are presented in Tables 5.7–5.9 of Chapter 5.

Table 4.13 further illustrates the variability within the population in *Producción de Palabras* [Words Produced]. As would be expected, at the younger months, a large majority of the children were reported to produce very few words. For instance, at 8 months of age, 51% of the sample were reported to not yet produce any words, and 42% of the sample were reported to produce between 1 and 10 words. With development, however, fewer children were reported to produce no words at all, and several of the 12-month-olds had more than 50 words. By 18 months of age, all of the children were reported to produce at least one word, with most children producing between 21 and 50 words. No child in the sample approached the ceiling value of 428 words.

Figure 4.7 presents the mean reported *Producción de Palabras* [Words Produced] scores by age and sex. Results of a 2 (sex) × 11 (age) between-subjects analysis of variance for vocabulary production revealed only a significant main effect of age, $F(10, 756) = 15.83$, $p < .01$. There was no significant main effect of sex, $F(1, 756) = 2.40$, *ns*, and no significant age × sex interaction, $F(10, 756) = 1.6$, *ns*. Age accounted for 17% of the variance. These results suggest similar overall levels of vocabulary and a generally upward developmental trajectory for both boys and girls.

***Gestos y Acciones* [Actions and Gestures]** Based on the responses in the *Gestos y Acciones* [Actions and Gestures] section, the mean *Total de Gestos* [Total Gestures] score (maximum = 64) for both sexes combined at each month is shown in Figure 4.8. Similar to the trend observed for *Comprensión de Palabras* [Words Understood], mean gesture usage tended to increase monotonically from 8 to 17 months but appeared to reach a slight plateau at 17 months. The variation remained relatively constant except at 8 months of age, where there appeared to be some reduction in the range of scores.

Table 4.14 provides further descriptive statistics for *Total de Gestos* [Total Gestures] as a function of age in months. Total scores averaged about 13 gestures at 8 months and increased to about 44 gestures, on average, by 18 months. These means are very similar to those reported for the English-speaking sam-

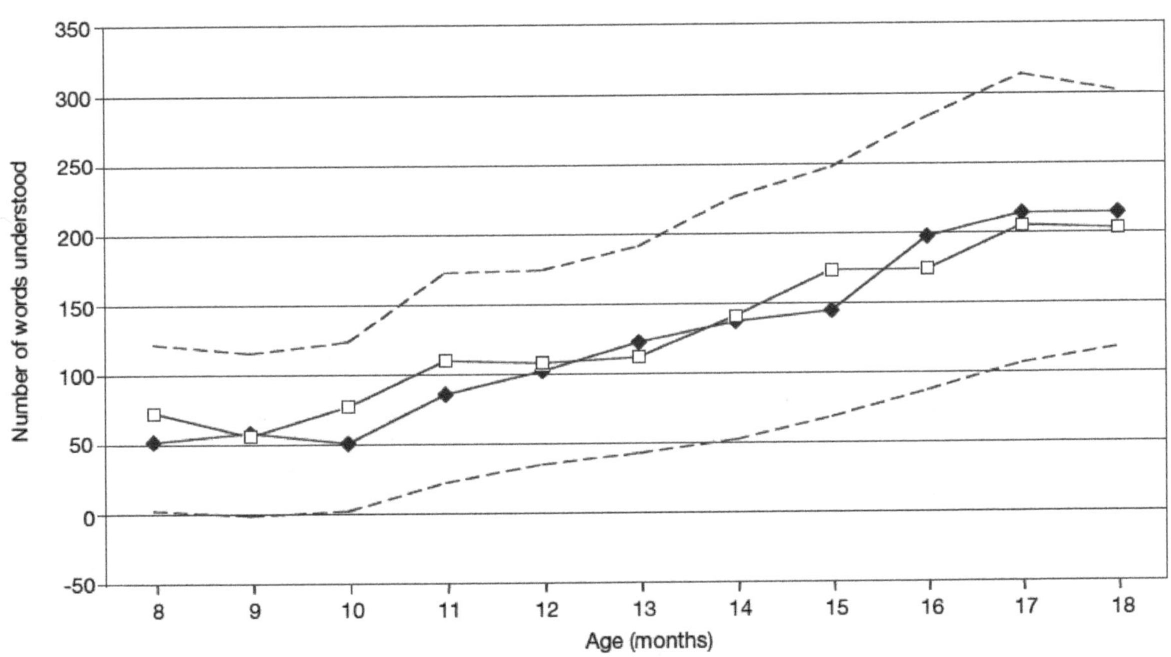

Figure 4.5. Mean *Comprensión de Palabras* [Words Understood] (Inventario I) scores by age and sex. (*Note:* The dashed lines represent ±1 standard deviation for the sexes combined.) (*Key:* —◆— boys; —□— girls.)

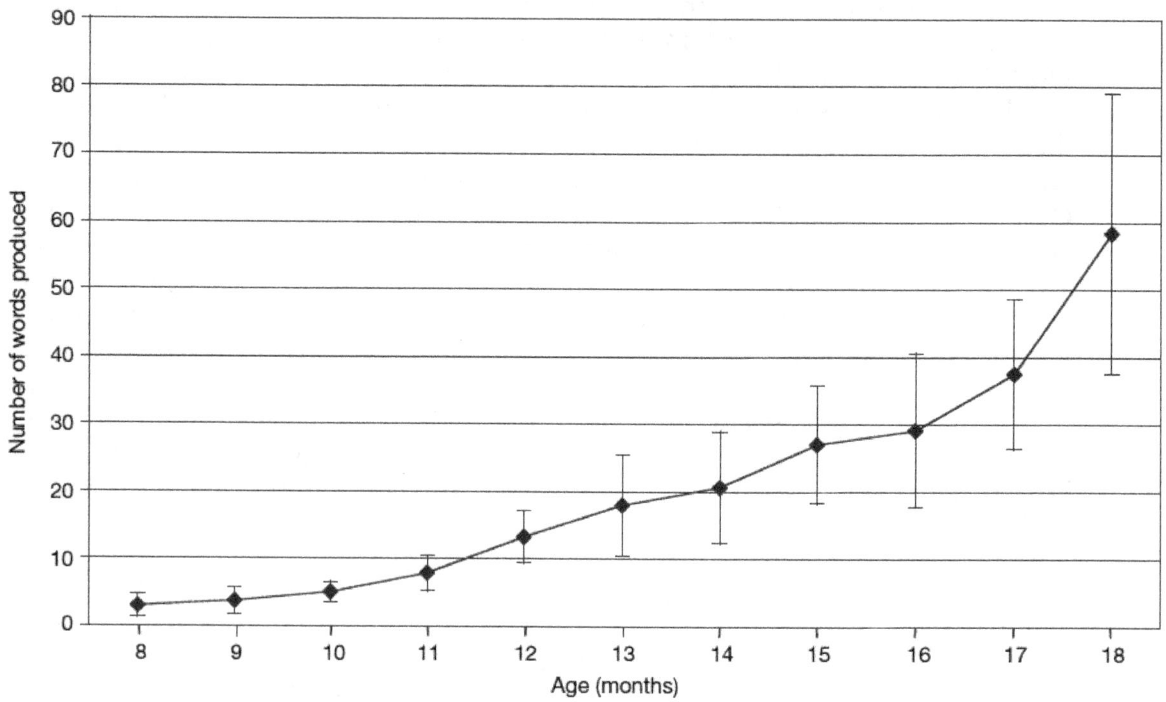

Figure 4.6. Mean *Producción de Palabras* [Words Produced] (Inventario I) scores by age in months. (*Note:* Bars above and below each mean score represent the 95.5% confidence intervals.)

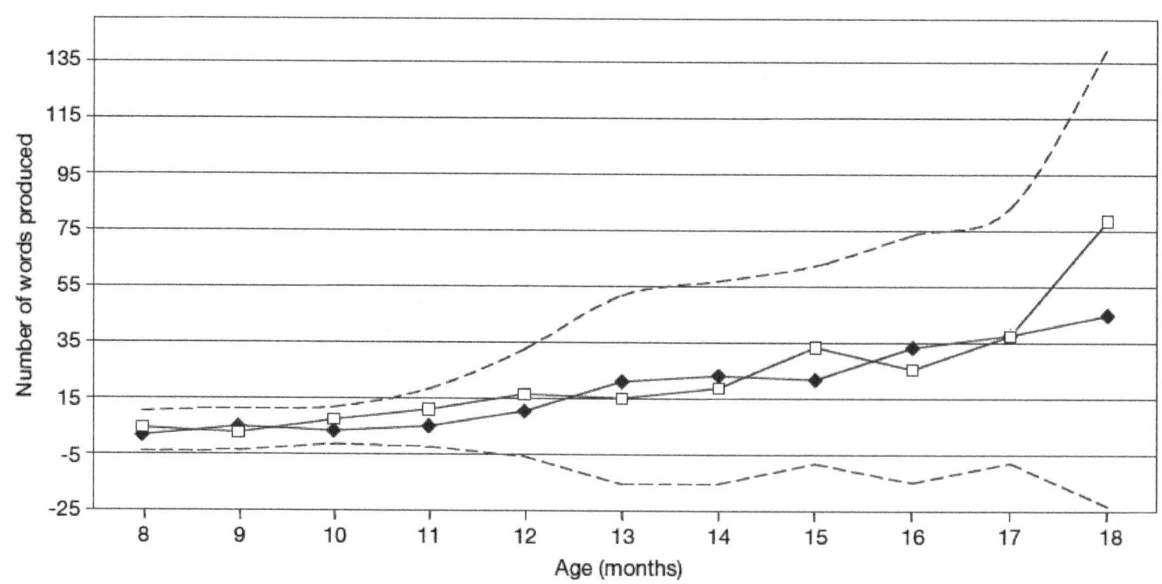

Figure 4.7. Mean *Producción de Palabras* [Words Produced] (Inventario I) scores by age and sex. (*Note:* The dashed lines represent ±1 standard deviation for the sexes combined.) (*Key:* —◆— boys; —□— girls.)

Table 4.12. Descriptive statistics for *Producción de Palabras* [Words Produced] (Inventario I)

Age in months	*n*	Mean	Median	Standard deviation	Minimum	Maximum[a]
8	71	3.0	0.0	7.1	0	48
9	59	3.7	1.0	7.5	0	43
10	77	5.0	3.0	6.6	0	33
11	65	7.8	3.0	10.4	0	49
12	96	13.2	7.0	19.1	0	91
13	80	18.0	8.0	33.5	0	231
14	75	20.6	8.0	36.1	0	228
15	66	27.0	12.0	35.2	0	179
16	60	29.2	12.5	44.1	0	274
17	67	37.5	20.0	45.5	0	206
18	62	58.3	25.0	81.6	1	351

[a]Maximum score possible = 428.

Table 4.13. Percentage of children with *Producción de Palabras* [Words Produced] (Inventario I) scores falling in five successive ranges

Age in months	*Producción de Palabras* [Words Produced][a]					
	0	1–10	11–20	21–50	51–100	> 100
8	50.7	42.3	4.2	2.8	0	0
9	40.7	50.8	5.1	3.4	0	0
10	32.5	55.8	6.5	5.2	0	0
11	30.8	43.1	15.4	10.8	0	0
12	15.6	49.0	19.8	6.3	9.4	0
13	13.8	43.8	22.5	13.8	2.5	3.8
14	13.3	48.0	14.7	12.0	8.0	4.0
15	6.1	42.4	16.7	16.7	12.1	6.1
16	10.0	30.0	26.7	13.3	15.0	5.0
17	4.5	26.9	19.4	28.4	10.4	10.4
18	0	24.2	12.9	32.3	16.1	14.5

[a]Maximum score possible = 428.

ple (see Figure 4-5 on p. 61 of Fenson et al., 1992/1993). As with the other measures, the range of scores was considerable throughout the age range. The percentile tables for this measure are Tables 5.10–5.12 in Chapter 5.

The variability in *Total de Gestos* [Total Gestures] scores can be further examined in Table 4.15. Early on (8–10 months), at least one child at each age level was reported to produce no gestures, whereas a few children had scores representing half of the possible items. From 16 to 18 months, several children approached the ceiling score of 64 gestures, yet a few children remained in the under-20 gesture range.

Total de Gestos [Total Gestures] for boys and girls at each age is plotted in Figure 4.9 as mean number of gestures. These scores were evaluated using a 2 (sex) × 11 (age) between-subjects analysis of variance. There was a significant main effect of sex, $F(1, 756) = 13.4, p < .001$, and a significant main effect of age, $F(10, 756) = 73.0, p < .001$. The sex × age interaction was not significant, $F(10, 756) = 1.0$, *ns*. Age accounted for 49% of the variance, and sex accounted for 2%

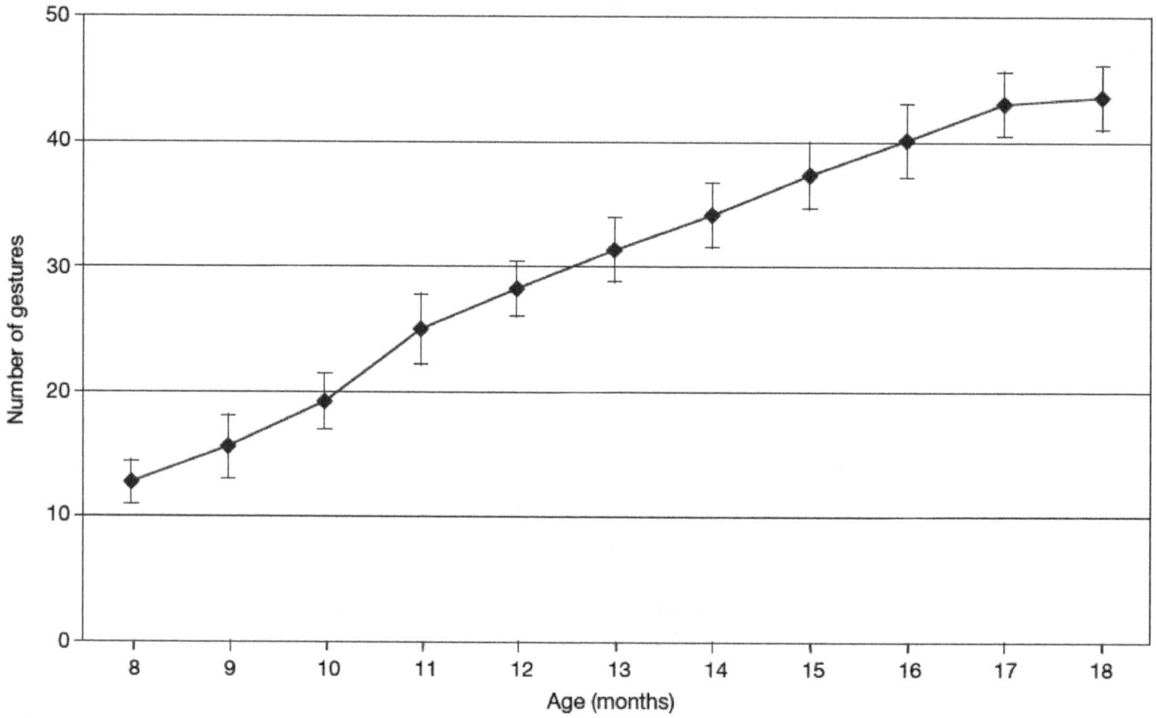

Figure 4.8. Mean *Total de Gestos* [Total Gestures] (Inventario I) scores by age in months. (*Note:* Bars below and above each mean score represent the 95.5% confidence intervals.)

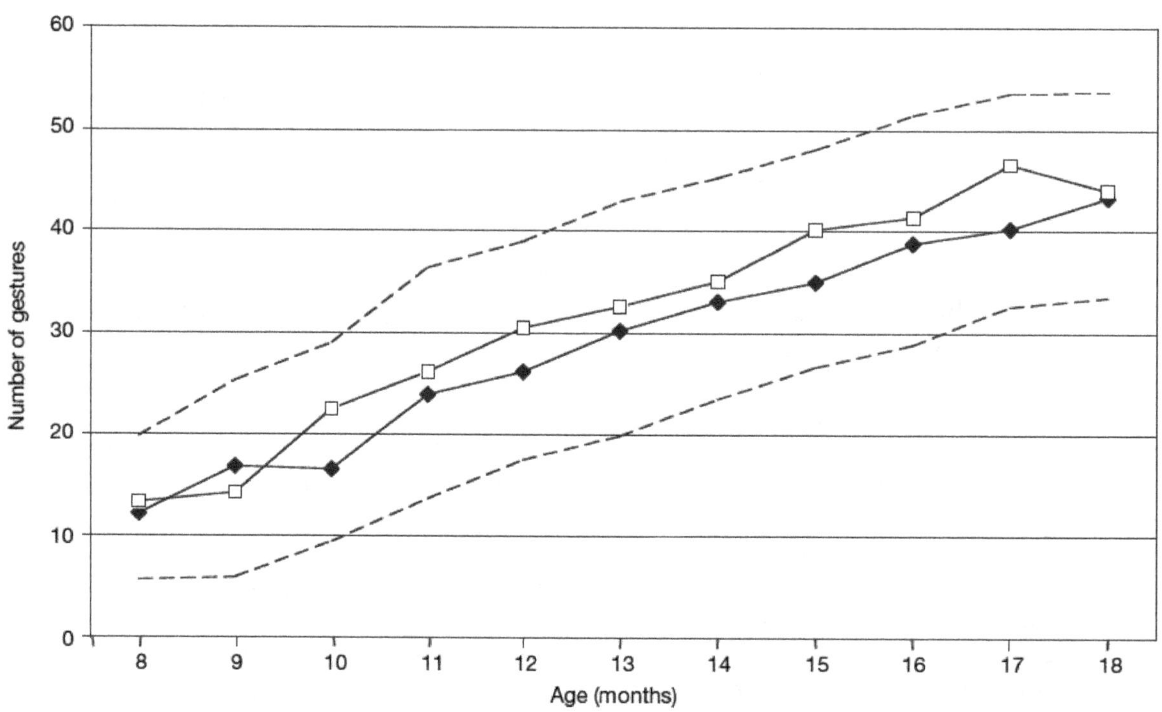

Figure 4.9. Mean *Total de Gestos* [Total Gestures] (Inventario I) scores reported by age and sex. (*Note:* The dashed lines represent ±1 standard deviation for the sexes combined.) (*Key:* —◆— boys; —□— girls.)

of the variance. As seen in Figure 4.9, the mean differences contributing to a significant main effect of sex result from higher gesture scores for girls than for boys, except at 9 and 18 months of age. To further evaluate this effect, individual t-test comparisons were performed with a modified Bonferroni correction. Results indicated that none of the 11 pair-wise comparisons were significant, suggesting that sex is a relatively minor contributor to differences across individuals in the frequency of reported gesture use in this age range.

Table 4.16 presents descriptive statistics for two gesture subcategories, *Gestos Tempranos* [Early Gestures] (the sum of Sections A and B of *Gestos y Acciones* [Actions and Gestures]) and *Gestos Tardíos* [Later Gestures] (the sum of Sections C through E of *Gestos y Acciones* [Actions and Gestures]). Consistent with findings on the English CDI, items composing the *Gestos Tempranos* [Early Gestures] subsection are more likely to be reported than items in the *Gestos Tardíos* [Later Gestures] sections, especially prior to 14 months of age. On average, children were reported to produce half of the *Gestos Tempranos* [Early Gestures] by 10 months of age, whereas half of the possible *Gestos*

Table 4.14. Descriptive statistics for *Total de Gestos* [Total Gestures] (Inventario I)

Age in months	*n*	Mean	Median	Standard deviation	Minimum	Maximum[a]
8	71	12.7	11.0	7.1	0	32
9	59	15.6	14.0	9.7	0	39
10	77	19.2	18.0	9.8	0	45
11	65	25.0	24.0	11.4	3	54
12	96	28.2	26.0	10.8	11	58
13	80	31.4	31.0	11.5	4	63
14	75	34.2	34.0	11.1	10	57
15	66	37.4	39.0	10.8	4	58
16	60	40.2	40.5	11.3	18	61
17	67	43.1	43.0	10.5	19	62
18	62	43.6	44.0	10.1	20	64

[a]Maximum score possible = 64.

Table 4.15. Percentage of children with *Total de Gestos* [Total Gestures] (Inventario I) scores falling in seven successive ranges

Age in months	*Total de Gestos* [Total Gestures][a]						
	0	1–10	11–20	21–30	31–40	41–50	51–64
8	4.2	35.2	46.5	11.3	2.8	0	0
9	1.7	32.2	39.0	18.6	8.5	0	0
10	1.3	22.1	35.1	26.0	13.0	2.6	0
11	0	7.7	27.7	35.4	23.1	1.5	4.6
12	0	0	29.2	35.4	18.8	14.6	2.1
13	0	5.0	11.3	32.5	27.5	18.8	5.0
14	0	2.7	12.0	14.7	44.0	20.0	6.7
15	0	1.5	1.5	28.8	25.8	33.3	9.1
16	0	0	1.7	25.0	23.3	30.0	20.0
17	0	0	1.5	13.4	26.9	32.8	25.4
18	0	0	3.2	9.7	22.6	35.5	29.0

[a]Maximum score possible = 64.

Table 4.16. Descriptive statistics for *Gestos Tempranos* [Early Gestures] and *Gestos Tardíos* [Later Gestures] (Inventario I)

Age in months	*n*	*Gestos Tempranos*[a] [Early Gestures]			*Gestos Tardíos*[b] [Later Gestures]		
		Mean	Median	*SD*	Mean	Median	*SD*
8	71	39.0	39.4	16.6	10.6	8.1	9.7
9	59	46.3	48.5	20.2	13.6	9.0	14.7
10	77	53.7	55.7	19.6	18.5	15.6	15.5
11	65	62.9	64.5	18.6	27.5	26.1	19.5
12	96	65.6	65.3	15.0	33.6	30.2	19.6
13	80	67.9	69.8	18.6	39.8	37.2	20.2
14	75	70.2	73.1	19.6	45.2	43.7	18.9
15	66	72.9	74.3	15.0	51.4	51.9	19.1
16	60	76.0	78.6	16.4	56.4	57.5	20.1
17	67	79.4	81.7	14.3	61.4	60.2	18.8
18	62	80.7	83.3	15.1	62.0	64.0	19.4

[a]For *Gestos Tempranos* [Early Gestures], mean and median scores are reported as a percentage of 21 opportunities.

[b]For *Gestos Tardíos* [Later Gestures], mean and median scores are reported as a percentage of 43 opportunities.

Tardíos [Later Gestures] were not reported as produced until 15 months of age. At the same time, there is considerable variation in gestures reported in each of these two subsections throughout the age period. Furthermore, there is some suggestion that children are approaching ceiling levels of performance on the *Gestos Tempranos* [Early Gestures] section by 17 to 18 months of age. The percentile tables for this measure are Tables 5.13–5.18 of Chapter 5.

Inventario II Components

Developmental trends in communicative development for each of the components of Inventario II are presented in this section as they appear on the Inventario and on the *Informe del Niño/a* [Child Report Form]. As mentioned in Chapter 1, English glosses are provided in square brackets; an asterisk marks a section that does not have a counterpart on the CDI: Words and Sentences.

***Lista de Vocabulario* [Vocabulary Checklist]** Figure 4.10 presents *Producción de Palabras* [Words Produced] for both sexes combined for children 16–30 months of age as mean number of words produced. The scores reflect a gradual, monotonically increasing trend, with relatively stable variation across the age range. The average number of words produced reported by parents was approximately 75 at 16 months, increasing to approximately 397 words by 30 months.

Table 4.17 provides complete descriptive information for *Producción de Palabras* [Words Produced] for children at each of the ages. These results highlight the variability in the entire age range, with scores spanning the range of possible values at each age. At almost every month, some children were reported to produce only a few words, whereas others were credited with producing more than 400 words.

Interestingly, these Spanish-speaking toddlers, on average, were generally reported to produce fewer words than the children in the English-speaking norming sample (see Figure 4-7 on p. 54 in Fenson et al., 1992/1993). The higher scores for the English-speaking children may be indicative of the generally higher socioeconomic level of that group of children. (See Table 4.4 for a comparison of the English and Spanish norming populations and the subsection later in this chapter called "Maternal Education" for a discussion of the relationship between maternal education and vocabulary outcomes.)

Comparing *Producción de Palabras* [Words Produced] for 16-, 17-, and 18-month-olds on Inventario II with the means for the same index on Inventario I (see Tables 4.17 and 4.12, respectively), we note that the means were generally higher for the children in the Inventario II sample. This finding could be a consequence of the composition of the respective norming samples. Alternatively, it may result from the fact that the *Lista de Vocabulario* [Vocabulary Checklist] contains more words on Inventario II (680) than it does on Inventario I (428), providing parents with more words that may be in their child's expressive vocabularies. The first possibility seems unlikely given the similarity in demographic characteristics across the two samples (see Table 4.3). The second seems more plausible given that a similar result was observed with the English CDIs at the only age point that overlapped between the Words and Gestures and Words and Sentences forms (i.e., 16 months). Nevertheless, the dis-

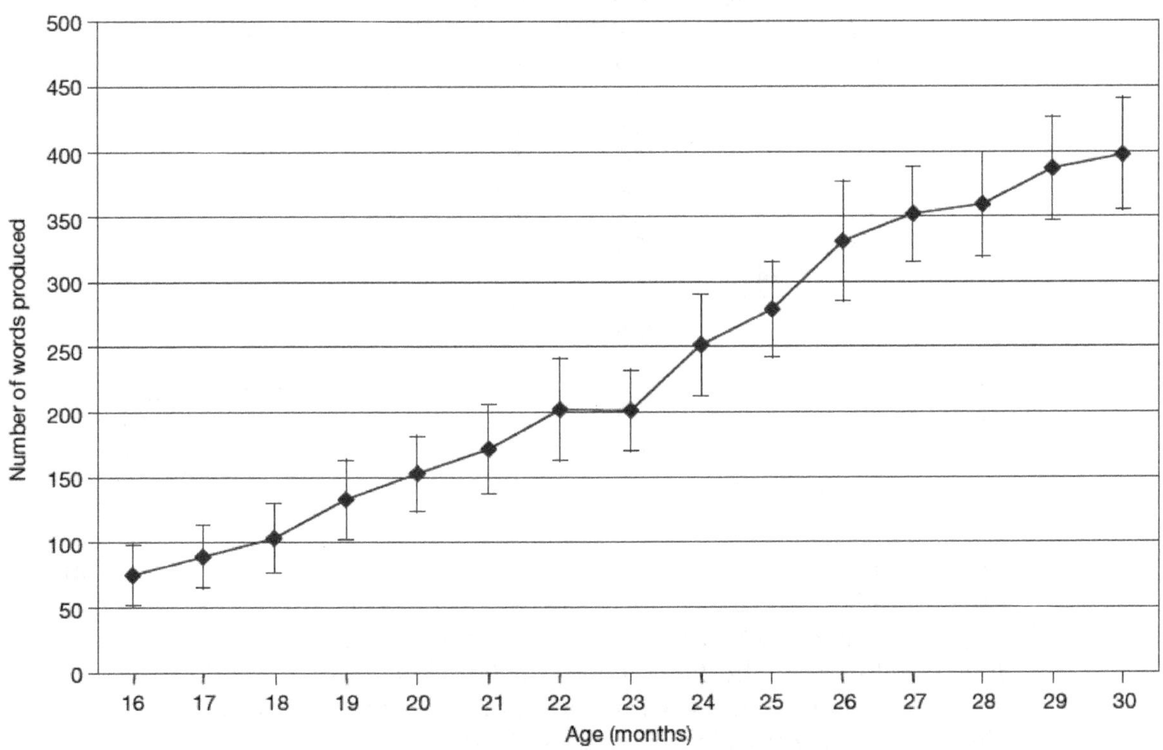

Figure 4.10. Mean *Producción de Palabras* [Words Produced] (Inventario II) scores by age in months. (*Note:* Bars below and above each mean score represent the 95.5% confidence intervals.)

Table 4.17. Descriptive statistics for *Producción de Palabras* [Words Produced] (Inventario II)

Age in months	*n*	Mean	Median	Standard deviation	Minimum	Maximum[a]
16	69	75.1	41.0	97.4	3	594
17	58	89.3	45.0	91.9	7	404
18	62	103.6	59.5	104.1	8	462
19	71	133.1	102.0	128.8	5	612
20	93	152.7	96.0	140.9	11	572
21	84	171.7	119.0	157.1	9	680
22	57	202.0	182.0	148.2	4	680
23	88	201.1	170.5	145.4	9	596
24	75	251.6	211.0	167.7	3	680
25	70	278.7	272.0	155.0	18	609
26	73	330.9	325.0	198.2	3	668
27	72	351.8	367.5	154.3	40	679
28	82	359.2	343.0	182.3	1	680
29	75	386.8	387.0	172.8	16	668
30	65	397.9	420.0	173.5	87	677

[a]Maximum score possible = 680.

Table 4.18. Percentage of children with *Producción de Palabras* [Words Produced] (Inventario II) scores falling in seven successive ranges

Age in months	*Producción de Palabras* [Words Produced][a]						
	0–100	101–200	201–300	301–400	401–500	501–600	601–680
16	75.4	15.9	5.8	1.4	0	1.4	0
17	67.2	20.7	6.9	3.4	1.7	0	0
18	66.1	17.7	9.7	3.2	3.2	0	0
19	49.3	26.8	15.5	4.2	1.4	1.4	1.4
20	50.5	21.5	12.9	5.4	7.5	2.2	0
21	42.9	22.6	19.0	7.1	2.4	2.4	3.6
22	29.8	22.8	22.8	14.0	8.8	0	1.8
23	31.8	26.1	13.6	19.3	5.7	3.4	0
24	18.7	28.0	17.3	16.0	10.7	4.0	5.3
25	17.1	18.6	21.4	24.3	5.7	10.0	2.9
26	15.1	13.7	19.2	15.1	13.7	9.6	13.7
27	4.2	13.9	22.2	16.7	25.0	11.1	6.9
28	8.5	11.0	22.0	15.9	15.9	13.4	13.4
29	6.7	10.7	12.0	24.0	17.3	17.3	12.0
30	1.5	13.8	20.0	10.8	23.1	15.4	15.4

[a]Maximum score possible = 680.

crepancies in absolute scores across the two forms serve as a reminder that the checklists provide indices of children's *relative* levels and should not be considered to provide an exhaustive atlas of a given child's vocabulary.

The variability in the *Producción de Palabras* [Words Produced] scores is further illustrated in Table 4.18 in terms of the proportion of children at each age who fall within 7 vocabulary ranges. At the youngest age (16 months), 75% of the sample was reported to produce between 0 and 100 words, and only one child was reported to produce more than 400 words. By 21 months, a majority of the children were reported to produce more than 100 words, although reported production vocabularies that were larger than 400 words were still relatively rare. By 30 months, slightly more than half of the children (approximately 54%) were reported to produce more than 400 words. At the same time, a few children were still reported to have production vocabularies of fewer than 100 words.

Producción de Palabras [Words Produced] for girls and boys at each age level is depicted in Figure 4.11 as mean number of words produced. Vocabulary production totals were analyzed with a 2 (sex) × 15 (age) between-subjects analysis of variance. This analysis yielded significant main effects of age, $F(14, 1{,}064) = 38.8$, $p < .01$, and sex, $F(1, 1{,}064) = 10.2$, $p < .01$, but a nonsignificant age × sex interaction, $F(14, 1{,}064) = 1.2$, *ns*. Age accounted for 34% of the variance, whereas sex accounted for only 1% of the variance. As seen in Figure 4.11, mean differences contributing to a significant main effect of sex are most apparent at the early (16–17 months) and later time points (26–30 months). Applying a modified Bonferroni correction ($p < .003$), individual t-test comparisons indicated that none of the 15 pair-wise comparisons were significant. Thus, sex is a relatively minor contributor to individual variation in reported production vocabulary levels for children in this sample. The percentile tables for boys and girls as well as for both sexes combined are Tables 5.19–5.21 in Chapter 5.

Cómo Usa y Comprende el Niño/a el Lenguaje **[How Children Use Words]** The section of Inventario II called *Cómo Usa y Comprende el Niño/a el Lenguaje* [How Children Use Words] consists of five items that assess the extent

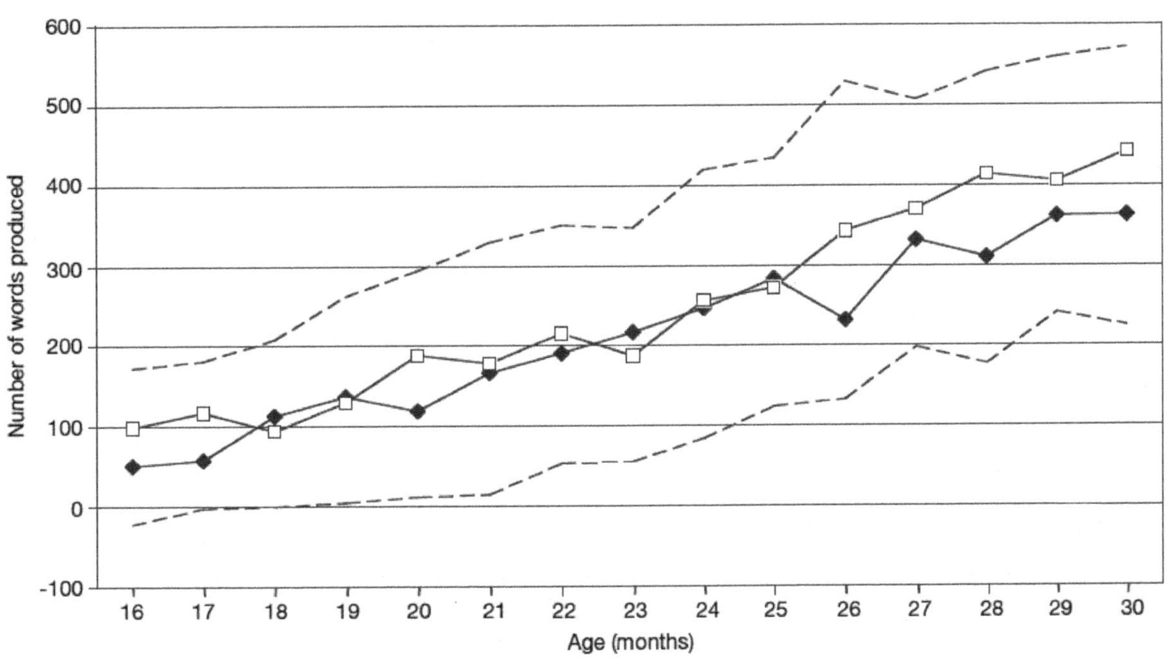

Figure 4.11. Mean *Producción de Palabras* [Words Produced] (Inventario II) scores by age and sex. (*Note:* The dashed lines represent ±1 standard deviation for the sexes combined.) (*Key:* —◆— boys; —□— girls.)

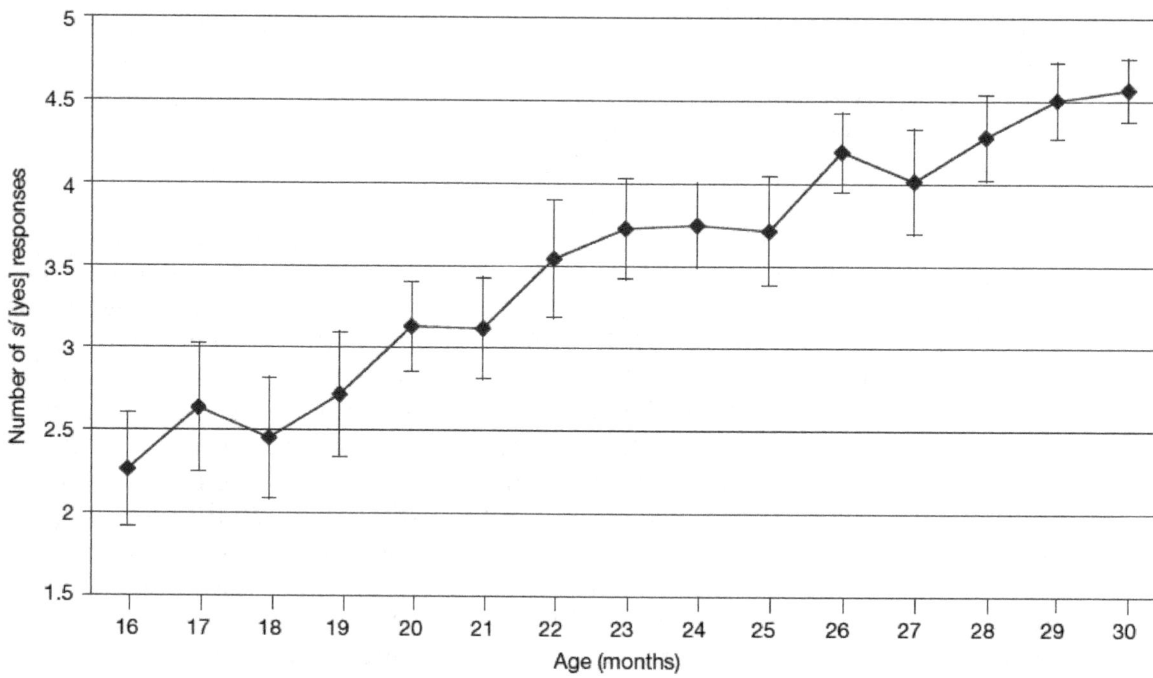

Figure 4.12. Mean *Cómo Usa y Comprende el Niño/a el Lenguaje* [How Children Use Words] (Inventario II) scores by age in months. (*Note:* Bars below and above each mean score represent the 95.5% confidence intervals.)

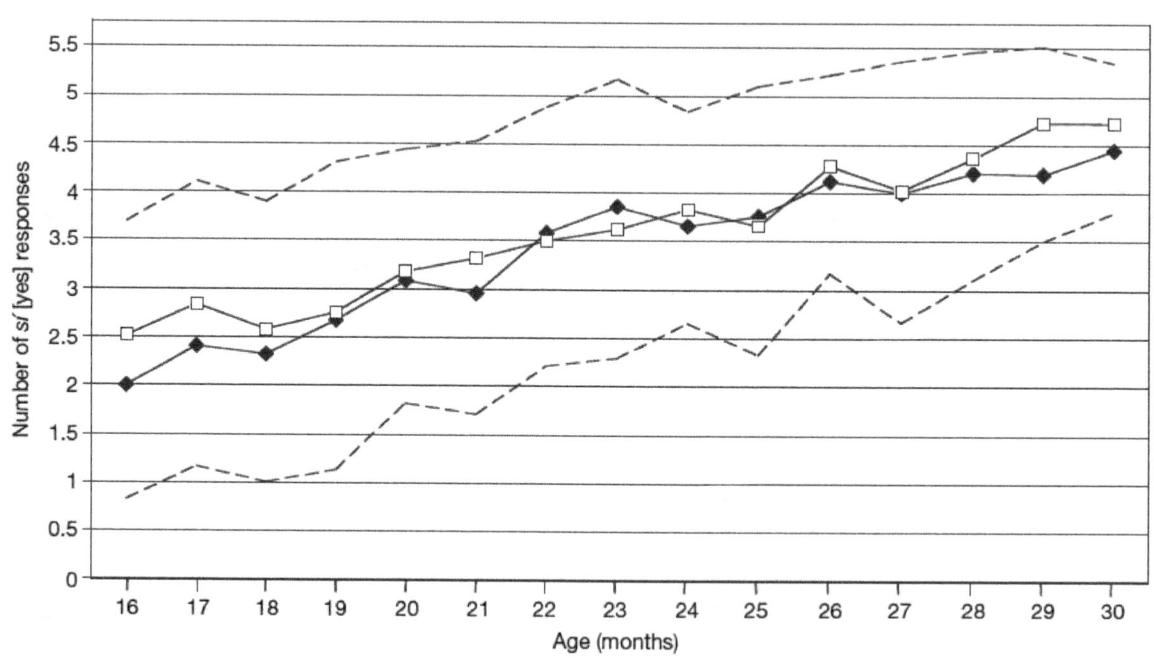

Figure 4.13. Mean *Cómo Usa y Comprende el Niño/a el Lenguaje* [How Children Use Words] (Inventario II) scores by age and sex. (*Note:* The dashed lines represent ±1 standard deviation for the sexes combined.) (*Key:* —◆— boys; —□— girls.)

Table 4.19. Descriptive statistics for *Cómo Usa y Comprende el Niño/a el Lenguaje* [How Children Use Words] (Inventario II)

Age in months	*n*	Mean	Median	Standard deviation	Minimum	Maximum[a]
16	69	2.3	2.0	1.4	0	5
17	58	2.6	3.0	1.5	0	5
18	62	2.4	2.5	1.4	0	5
19	71	2.7	3.0	1.6	0	5
20	93	3.1	3.0	1.3	0	5
21	84	3.1	3.0	1.4	0	5
22	57	3.5	4.0	1.3	0	5
23	88	3.7	4.0	1.4	0	5
24	75	3.8	4.0	1.1	1	5
25	70	3.7	4.0	1.4	0	5
26	73	4.2	5.0	1.0	1	5
27	72	4.0	4.5	1.4	0	5
28	82	4.3	5.0	1.2	0	5
29	75	4.5	5.0	1.0	0	5
30	65	4.6	5.0	0.8	2	5

[a]Maximum score posible = 5.

to which children use words to refer to the past or future or to missing or absent objects or people. The mean number of *sí* [yes] responses (5 possible) on this section by age in months is shown in Figure 4.12, and further descriptive information is provided in Table 4.19. We see that the mean number of responses increased over the 16- to 30-month period, demonstrating a generally monotonically increasing trend with age. Variation in scores was quite substantial, spanning the entire range of possible scores at each age. There is some suggestion that the variation tends to decrease in the later months.

The mean number of *sí* [yes] responses is presented for girls and boys separately at each age level in Figure 4.13. Totals on this measure were analyzed with a 2 (sex) × 15 (age) between-subjects analysis of variance. This analysis yielded significant main effects of age, $F(14, 1{,}064) = 39.0$, $p < .01$, and sex, $F(1, 1{,}064) = 8.2$, $p < .03$, but a nonsignificant age × sex interaction, $F(14, 1{,}064) = 0.5$, *ns*. Similar to other measures, mean differences contributing to a significant main effect of sex are most apparent at early (16–17 months) and later time points (26–30 months). At the same time, individual *t*-test comparisons indicated that none of the 15 pair-wise comparisons were significant ($p < .003$), suggesting a relatively minor contribution of sex to the individual variation that is observed in this measure.

Differences in the developmental pace of acquisition for the 5 items in this section are displayed in Table 4.20. These data indicate that references to the past and future emerged later than the comprehension and production of references to absent objects. A similar trend was found for English-speaking toddlers (see Table 4-11 on p. 56 in Fenson et al., 1992/1993). We should note, however, that the emergence of these uses of language, in general, occurred slightly later for Spanish-speaking infants than for their English-speaking counterparts.

***Formas de Verbos* [*Verb Forms]** The *Formas de Verbos* [*Verb Forms] section presents examples of three verb conjugations (*Presente* [*Present], *Pasado* [*Past], and *Imperativo* [*Imperative]) across three verb classes (*-ar, -er, -ir*). Figure 4.14 plots the mean number of verb forms (24 possible) reported to be produced as a function of age in months. The descriptive statistics for the total number of verb conjugation forms marked at each month are presented in Table 4.21. In general, the scores demonstrate a gradual, monotonically increasing trend. There is also wide variability on this scale. The variation in scores is somewhat larger in the later months than in the earlier age periods.

Table 4.22 presents the proportion of reported responses in each of the three subsections of *Formas de Verbos* [*Verb Forms]: *Presente* [*Present] (12 items), *Pasado* [*Past] (6 items), and *Imperativo* [*Imperative] (6 items). For comparability across sections, the data are presented as percentages of possible responses. These data indicate similar gradual, monotonically increasing trends and wide variability at each month for each of the three subcategories taken individually. When interpreting these results, it must be remembered that there are twice as many items in the category *Presente* [*Present] than in each of the other two categories.

***Combinación de Palabras* [Combining]** In the second part of Inventario II, parents were asked to indicate whether their child had begun to produce word combinations. Figure 4.15 presents the mean reported scores for this measure by age and sex, and Table 4.23 presents the percentage of girls and boys at each month with responses categorized as *todavía no* [not yet] or *sí* [yes] (*de vez en*

Table 4.20. Percentage of children with *sí* [yes] responses for items in *Cómo Usa y Comprende el Niño/a el Lenguaje* [How Children Use Words] (Inventario II)

	Cómo Usa y Comprende el Niño/a el Lenguaje [How Children Use Words]				
Age in months	*Pasado* [Past]	*Futuro* [Future]	*Objeto Ausente (Producción)* [Absent Object (Production)]	*Objeto Ausente (Comprensión)* [Absent Object (Comprehension)]	*Dueño Ausente* [Absent Owner]
16	17.4	18.8	60.9	82.6	46.4
17	20.7	29.3	72.4	87.9	53.4
18	17.7	19.4	69.4	83.9	54.8
19	25.4	29.6	69.0	87.3	60.6
20	29.0	33.3	84.9	93.5	72.0
21	34.5	33.3	77.4	96.4	70.2
22	50.9	40.4	89.5	94.7	78.9
23	55.7	51.1	90.9	93.2	81.8
24	50.7	53.3	93.3	93.3	84.0
25	61.4	48.6	88.6	92.9	80.0
26	72.6	64.4	95.9	97.3	89.0
27	68.1	65.3	90.3	90.3	87.5
28	72.0	74.4	92.7	96.3	92.7
29	84.0	82.7	96.0	94.7	93.3
30	86.2	81.5	92.3	98.5	98.5

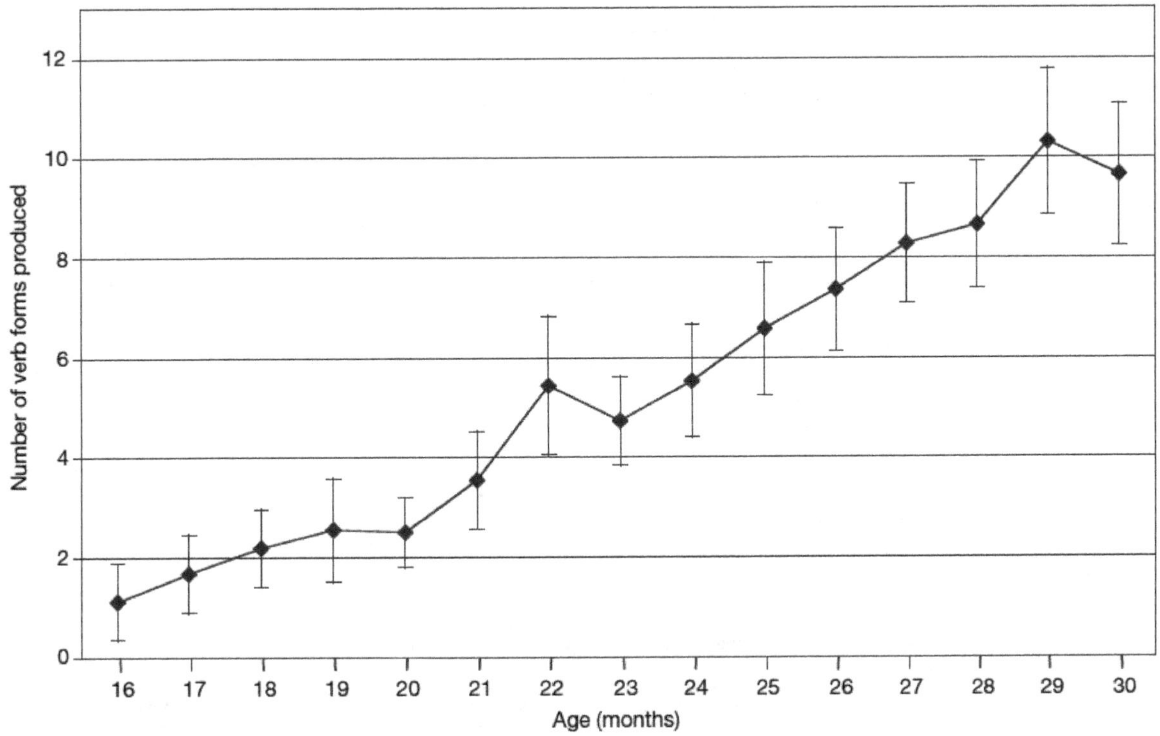

Figure 4.14. Mean *Formas de Verbos* [*Verb Forms] (Inventario II) scores by age in months. (*Note:* Bars below and above each mean score represent the 95.5% confidence intervals.)

cuando [sometimes] and *muchas veces* [often] combined). Results indicate that most children in the youngest age groups (16–18 months) were not likely to combine words. By 28 months, more than 80% of the sample was reported to produce word combinations, at least *de vez en cuando* [sometimes]. These results are generally similar to the English data (see Table 4-14 on p. 60 in Fenson et al., 1992/1993). In the English-speaking sample, however, all children were reported to combine words by 28 months. In the Spanish-speaking sample, in contrast, some parents of boys reported that their child did not combine words as late as 30 months of age.

Frequencies of combining were analyzed with a 2 (sex) × 15 (age) between-subjects analysis of variance. This analysis yielded significant main effects of age, $F(14, 1{,}064) = 20.8$, $p < .001$, and sex, $F(1, 1{,}064) = 8.7$, $p < .003$, but a nonsignificant age × sex interaction, $F(14, 1{,}064) = 0.9$, *ns*. Age accounted for 20% of the variance, whereas sex accounted for 0.8% of the variance. Table 4.23 indicates that the mean differences contributing to a significant main effect of sex are most apparent at the early (16–17 months) and to some extent, the later (28–30 months) ages. However, individual *t*-test comparisons using a modified Bonferroni correction ($p < .003$) indicated that none of the 15 pair-wise comparisons were significant. Thus, sex differences are observed in this measure but must be considered to be a relatively minor contributor to the overall variation in scores.

Table 4.21. Descriptive statistics for *Formas de Verbos* [*Verb Forms] (Inventario II)

Age in months	*n*	Mean	Median	Standard deviation	Minimum	Maximum[a]
16	69	1.1	0.0	3.2	0	24
17	58	1.7	0.0	3.0	0	14
18	62	2.2	0.0	3.1	0	12
19	71	2.5	1.0	4.4	0	24
20	93	2.5	1.0	3.4	0	16
21	84	3.5	2.0	4.5	0	24
22	57	5.4	4.0	5.2	0	24
23	88	4.7	4.0	4.2	0	17
24	75	5.5	4.0	4.9	0	24
25	70	6.6	5.5	5.6	0	23
26	73	7.4	7.0	5.2	0	22
27	72	8.3	8.5	5.1	0	23
28	82	8.7	9.0	5.8	0	24
29	75	10.3	9.0	6.4	0	24
30	65	9.7	9.0	5.7	0	24

[a]Maximum score possible = 24.

Table 4.22. Descriptive statistics for subclasses of *Formas de Verbos* [*Verb Forms] (Inventario II)

Age in months	*n*	*Presente* [*Present][a] Mean (%)	*SD*	*Pasado* [*Past][b] Mean (%)	*SD*	*Imperativo* [*Imperative][b] Mean (%)	*SD*
16	69	5.0	13.9	3.6	13.4	5.1	14.4
17	58	7.0	11.3	6.9	15.3	6.9	15.9
18	62	8.6	12.5	8.6	15.9	10.8	17.4
19	71	11.0	19.5	11.0	19.7	9.4	19.9
20	93	9.7	13.7	11.6	18.0	10.8	19.5
21	84	14.2	17.9	15.3	21.8	15.5	23.1
22	57	20.2	21.1	26.3	27.8	24.0	26.2
23	88	18.7	17.1	20.8	24.3	20.6	21.4
24	75	21.8	20.0	26.4	27.3	22.2	23.9
25	70	24.8	22.5	31.9	28.8	28.1	28.2
26	73	27.3	24.8	37.7	26.5	30.4	25.2
27	72	32.5	22.4	40.3	27.5	32.6	24.0
28	82	32.1	27.4	42.7	30.0	37.4	26.1
29	75	38.7	28.2	52.9	30.7	41.8	28.4
30	65	34.7	25.5	51.0	29.7	40.5	27.3

[a]12 items possible.
[b]6 items possible.

***Ejemplos* [Examples]** Parents who indicated that their child had begun to combine words were asked to write the three longest utterances that they had recently heard their child say. The mean of the three longest utterances in words (*M3L-Palabras* [M3L-*Words]) was computed by adding the number of words in each utterance and dividing by the number of utterances provided. In a few cases ($n = 26$, 2.4%), the parent indicated that his or her child had begun to combine words but did not offer any examples. In these cases, the score was reported as missing data. If the parent did not report that the child was combining words but filled in the utterances, the scores for *Combinación de Palabras* [Combining] indicate that the child was combining words. The same was done if the parent did not report that the child was combining words but filled in the *Complejidad de Frases* [Complexity] section. In each case the scores for *M3L-Palabras* [M3L-*Words] and *Complejidad de Frases* [Complexity] were calculated and used.

Figure 4.16 presents the average *M3L-Palabras* [M3L-*Words] scores as a function of age. On average, the length of the reported utterances for this sample of toddlers was fairly short, approximately 1.5 words at the earliest ages. The reported longest utterances, however, increased to a mean of about 5 words by 30 months of age. Note that the variation in range of scores is considerably smaller during the early months than the later ages due to the fact that at the earlier months the majority of the children in the sample were not yet reported to produce word combinations.

Table 4.24 presents more complete descriptive statistics for *M3L-Palabras* [M3L-*Words]. As with the other measures, *M3L-Palabras* [M3L-*Words] shows wide variability, especially at the older ages. Overall growth in this measure was monotonic, with mean scores increasing steadily across the age period. Direct numerical comparison cannot be made between the Spanish and English M3L mean scores because of differences in the computational methods used to determine the mean length of each utterance indicated by the parent. English M3L scores were based on the number of morphemes in each utterance. In con-

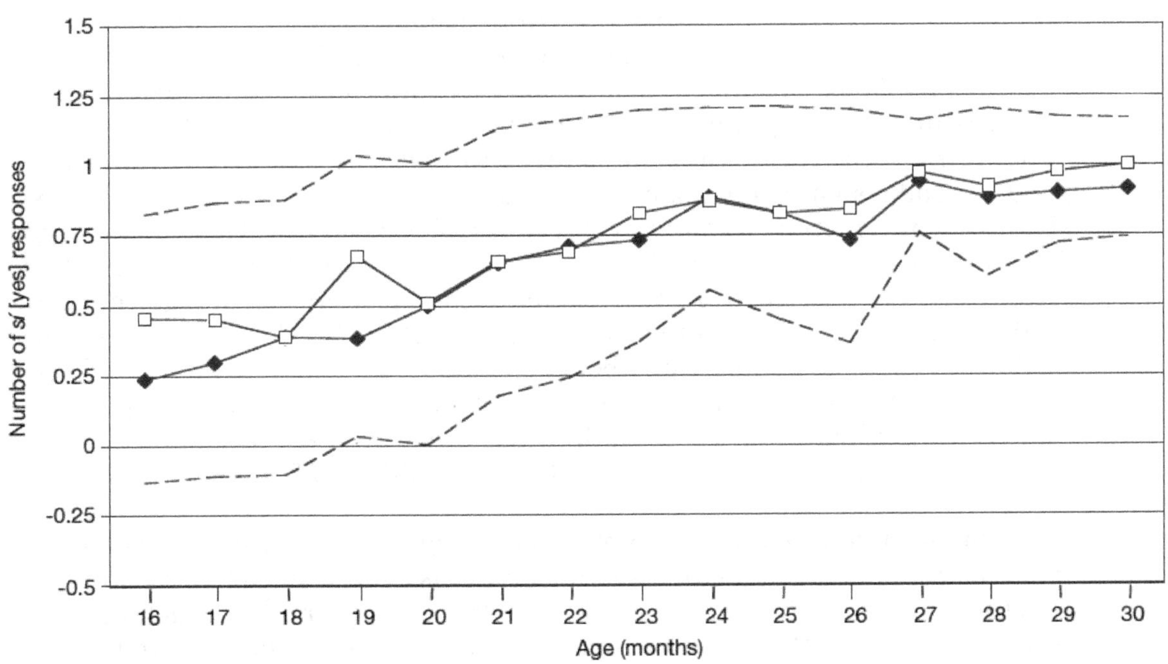

Figure 4.15. Mean *Combinación de Palabras* [Combining] (Inventario II) scores by age and sex. (*Note:* The dashed lines represent ±1 standard deviation for the sexes combined.) (*Key:* —◆— boys; —□— girls.)

Table 4.23. Percentage of children with *sí* [yes] responses on *Combinación de Palabras* [Combining] (Inventario II)

	Girls		Boys	
Age in months	*todavía no* [not yet]	*sí* [yes]	*todavía no* [not yet]	*sí* [yes]
16	54.3	45.7	76.5	23.5
17	54.8	45.2	70.4	29.6
18	61.3	38.7	61.3	38.7
19	32.4	67.6	61.8	38.2
20	48.9	51.1	50.0	50.0
21	34.2	65.8	34.8	65.2
22	30.8	69.2	29.0	71.0
23	17.0	83.0	26.8	73.2
24	12.5	87.5	11.4	88.6
25	17.2	82.8	17.1	82.9
26	15.6	84.4	26.8	73.2
27	2.6	97.4	5.9	94.1
28	7.7	92.3	11.6	88.4
29	2.3	97.7	9.7	90.3
30	0	100.0	8.3	91.7

trast, words were used as the unit for calculating the mean length of each utterance for Spanish because there is disagreement about how to derive a simple numerical count of morphemes in a morphologically rich language such as Spanish (Gutiérrez-Clellen et al., 2000). An M3L calculated using words results in a lower mean score than an M3L calculated using morphemes. Consequently, one would expect the Spanish scores to be generally lower than the English scores, and this is the case (see Figure 4-12 on p. 61 in Fenson et al., 1993).

Figure 4.17 presents mean *M3L-Palabras* [M3L-*Words] scores for boys and girls in each age group. A 2 (sex) × 15 (age) between-subjects analysis of variance for M3L yielded a significant main effect of sex, $F(1, 1{,}038) = 24.2$, $p < .001$, and a significant main effect of age, $F(14, 1{,}038) = 39.0$, $p < .001$. No significant interaction was found, $F(14, 1{,}038) = 1.44$, *ns*. Age accounted for 34.5% of the variance, and sex accounted for 2% of the variance. Modified Bonferroni tests were used to further evaluate the apparent advantage that girls held over boys that contributed to the significant main effect. However, none of the 15 pair-wise comparisons between the mean scores for boys and girls were significant, suggesting that sex is not a reliable and substantive predictor of the variation that is observed in this measure. The percentile tables for boys and girls as well as for both sexes combined are Tables 5.22–5.24 in Chapter 5.

***Complejidad de Frases* [Complexity]** Each of the 37 items in the *Complejidad de Frases* [Complexity] section contains a more and a less complicated phrase or sentence. Parents were asked to mark the example in each pair that sounded more like the way in which their child speaks. The *Complejidad de Frases* [Complexity] score represents the number of times the parents selected the more complex example of the pair (37 maximum). Figure 4.18 presents mean complexity scores by age in months, and Table 4.25 provides an overview of the descriptive statistics for complexity. As would be expected, children were more likely to be reported to sound like the more complex examples as they increased in age from 16 to 30 months, with a somewhat more rapid trajectory after about 24 months. In addition, there is considerably less variation in the scores during the early period, when fewer children are reported to be producing word combinations. This trend is similar to that observed in the English norming study up to about 20 months of age. After this time, scores on this measure as reported in the English norms are slightly higher (see Figure 4-13 on p. 62 of Fenson et al., 1992/1993).

Tables 4.25 and 4.26 further highlight the changes in mean complexity scores, including the wide distribution of scores. At every month, at least one child who was reported to be producing word combinations was reported to not use the more complex form of any of the example sentence pairs. From 19 months on, though, one or more children at each age was at or near the maximum score of 37. As for most measures, mean scores were lower (after 20 months) for the Spanish-speaking than for the English-speaking sample (see Figure 4-13 on p. 62 in Fenson et al., 1992/1993). The majority of children up to 23 months of age did not use the more complex form of the examples provided in this section of Inventario II. By 27 months, a majority of the children were credited with at least some use of the more complex forms.

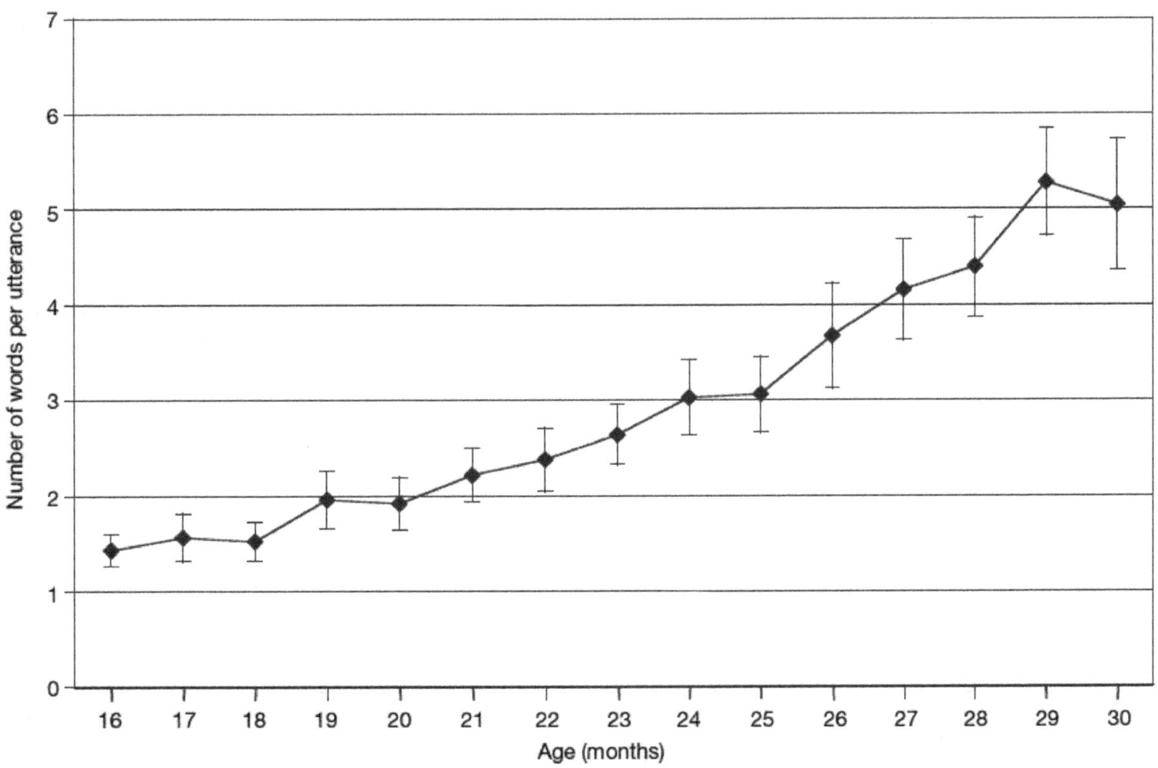

Figure 4.16. Mean *M3L-Palabras* [M3L-*Words] (Inventario II) scores by age in months. (*Note:* Bars below and above each mean score represent the 95.5% confidence intervals.)

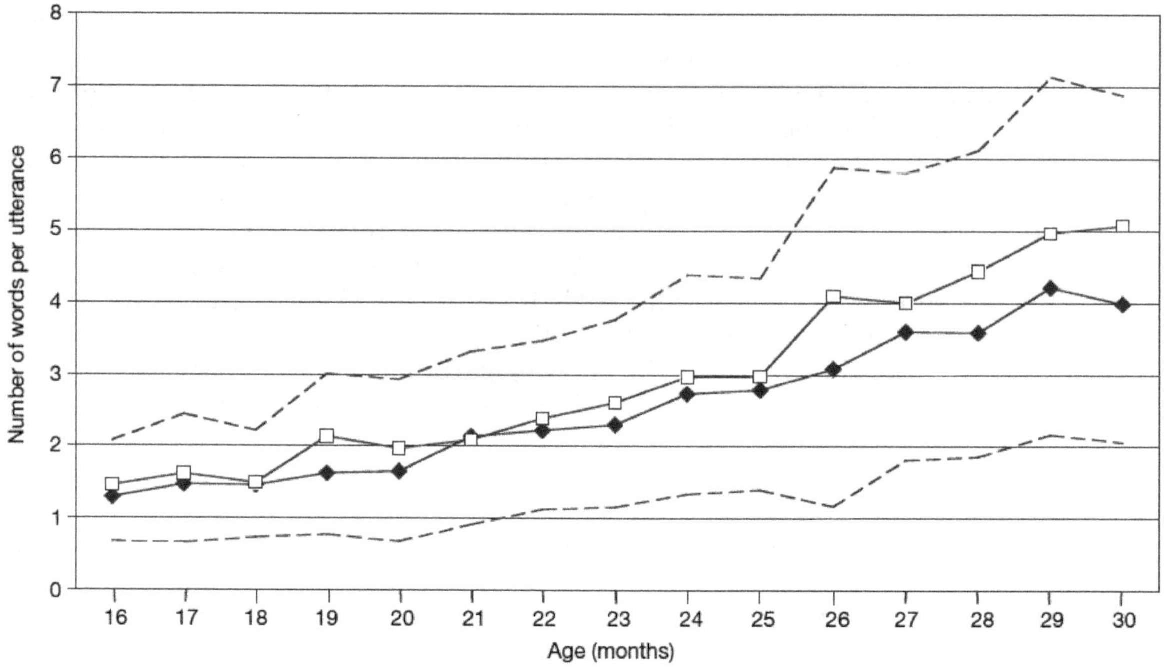

Figure 4.17. Mean *M3L-Palabras* [M3L-*Words] (Inventario II) scores by age and sex. (*Note:* The dashed lines represent ±1 standard deviation for the sexes combined.) (*Key:* —◆— boys; —□— girls.)

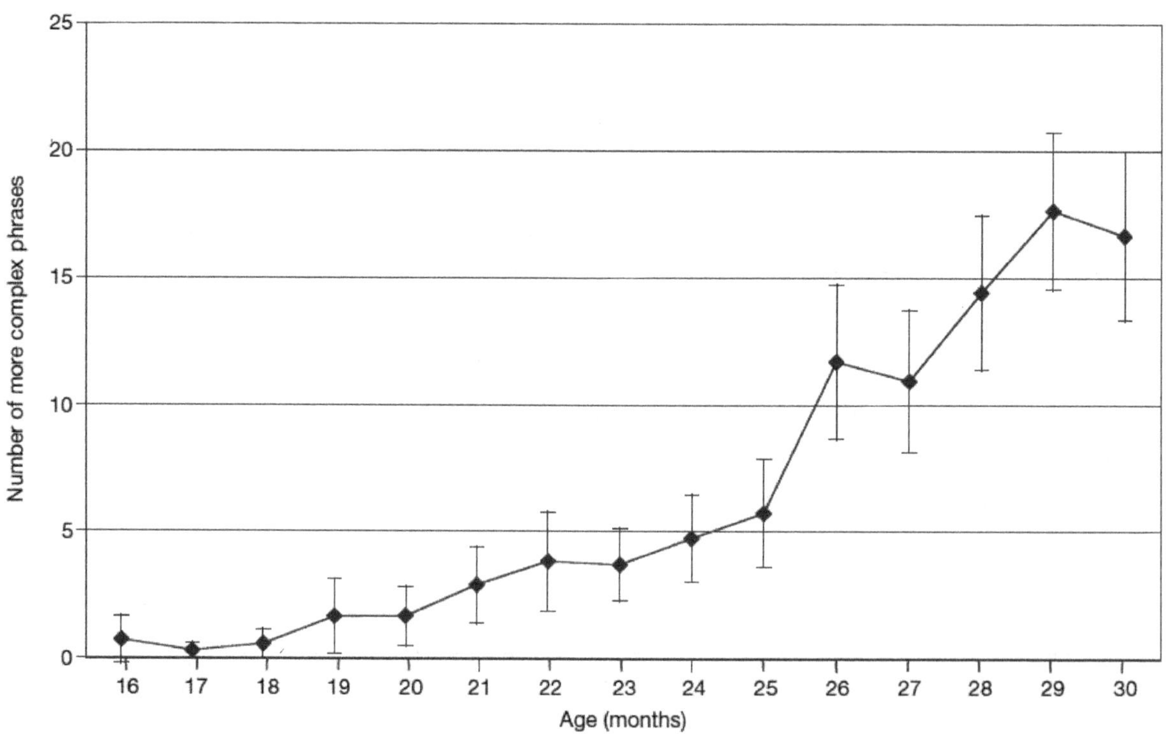

Figure 4.18. Mean *Complejidad de Frases* [Complexity] (Inventario II) scores by age in months. (*Note:* Bars below and above each mean score represent the 95.5% confidence intervals.)

Table 4.24. Descriptive statistics for *M3L-Palabras* [M3L-*Words] (Inventario II)

Age in months	*n*	Mean	Median	Standard deviation	Minimum	Maximum
16	69	1.4	1.0	0.7	1.0	4.0
17	58	1.6	1.0	0.9	1.0	5.3
18	62	1.5	1.0	0.8	1.0	4.3
19	71	2.0	1.7	1.2	1.0	7.0
20	92	1.9	1.4	1.3	1.0	10.0
21	85	2.2	2.0	1.3	1.0	6.7
22	57	2.4	2.3	1.2	1.0	6.7
23	88	2.6	2.3	1.5	1.0	8.7
24	75	3.0	3.0	1.7	1.0	10.0
25	70	3.1	3.0	1.6	1.0	9.3
26	73	3.7	3.3	2.4	1.0	12.3
27	72	4.2	3.6	2.2	1.0	10.3
28	82	4.4	4.3	2.4	1.0	12.7
29	75	5.3	5.3	2.4	1.0	12.0
30	65	5.1	4.7	2.7	1.0	12.0

For both of the grammatical measures, *Complejidad de Frases* [Complexity] and *M3L-Palabras* [M3L-*Words], the scores for the 30-month-old group are equivalent to or lower than the scores for the 29-month-olds. This is not a result of ceiling effects. The M3L score has no ceiling, and the top score of 37 for the sentence complexity items far exceeds the 29- and 30-month mean scores of 17 and 16, respectively. The effect is presumably due to sampling variation and is minimized by the curve-fitting procedures used to determine the percentile scores in Tables 5.25–5.27 in Chapter 5.

Mean scores for *Complejidad de Frases* [Complexity] for boys and girls at each age are shown in Figure 4.19. Results from a 2 (sex) × 15 (age) between-subjects analysis of variance yielded a significant main effect of sex, $F(1, 1{,}064) = 10.94$, $p < .01$, and a significant main effect of age, $F(14, 1{,}064) = 32.09$, $p < .01$, but no significant interaction, $F(14, 1{,}064) = 1.33$, *ns.* Age accounted for 30% of the variance, whereas sex accounted for 1%. Modified Bonferroni tests were used to further evaluate the main effect of sex. As we have seen in the other measures, none of the 15 pair-wise comparisons were significant ($p < .003$), suggesting only a minor impact of sex on the variability of the scores from this measure.

IMPACT OF DEMOGRAPHIC FACTORS ON LANGUAGE OUTCOMES

Maternal Education

Maternal education was adopted as an index of socioeconomic status (SES) for two reasons. First, it is more easily and reliably obtained than other indices of SES, such as family income. Second, it has traditionally been found to be a strong correlate of other measures of SES (Dollaghan et al., 1999; Garcia Coll,

1990; Jackson-Maldonado et al., 1993; Laosa, 1982; Walker, Greenwood, Hart, & Carta, 1994). Hart and Risley (1995) reported that SES based on occupation was more strongly correlated with the education of both parents ($r = .86$) than with maternal education alone ($r = .73$), but both correlations are strong. For the analyses described here, maternal education was divided into three levels: no school, some high school, and some college. The sample for Inventario I was divided into two age periods (8–12 months and 13–18 months). The Inventario II sample was divided into three age periods (16–20 months, 21–25 months, and 26–30 months). This grouping strategy ensured that there were a sufficient

Table 4.25. Descriptive statistics for *Complejidad de Frases* [Complexity] (Inventario II)

Age in months	*n*	Mean	Median	Standard deviation	Minimum	Maximum[a]
16	69	0.7	0.1	3.9	0	31
17	58	0.3	0.1	1.1	0	7
18	62	0.6	0.1	2.2	0	11
19	71	1.7	0.3	6.2	0	36
20	93	1.7	0.3	5.6	0	37
21	84	2.9	0.6	7.0	0	37
22	57	3.8	0.8	7.4	0	37
23	88	3.7	0.8	6.8	0	33
24	75	4.8	1.7	7.4	0	36
25	70	5.7	1.3	8.9	0	37
26	73	11.7	5.8	13.0	0	37
27	72	10.9	5.3	11.9	0	36
28	82	14.4	9.7	13.9	0	37
29	75	17.7	16.2	13.4	0	37
30	65	16.7	14.0	13.4	0	37

[a]Maximum score possible = 37.

Table 4.26. Percentage of children at each age with *Complejidad de Frases* [Complexity] (Inventario II) scores falling in four successive ranges

Age in months	*Complejidad de Frases* [Complexity] scores[a]			
	0	1–10	11–20	21–37
16	89.9	8.7	0	1.4
17	89.7	10.3	0	0
18	87.1	11.3	1.6	0
19	73.2	22.5	1.4	2.8
20	75.3	19.4	2.2	3.2
21	56.0	36.9	2.4	4.8
22	52.6	35.1	8.8	3.5
23	51.1	38.6	5.7	4.5
24	40.0	44.0	10.7	5.3
25	41.4	38.6	11.4	8.6
26	34.2	21.9	16.4	27.4
27	9.7	55.6	11.1	23.6
28	24.4	26.8	14.6	34.1
29	13.3	26.7	18.7	41.3
30	13.8	24.6	20.0	41.5

[a]Maximum score possible= 37.

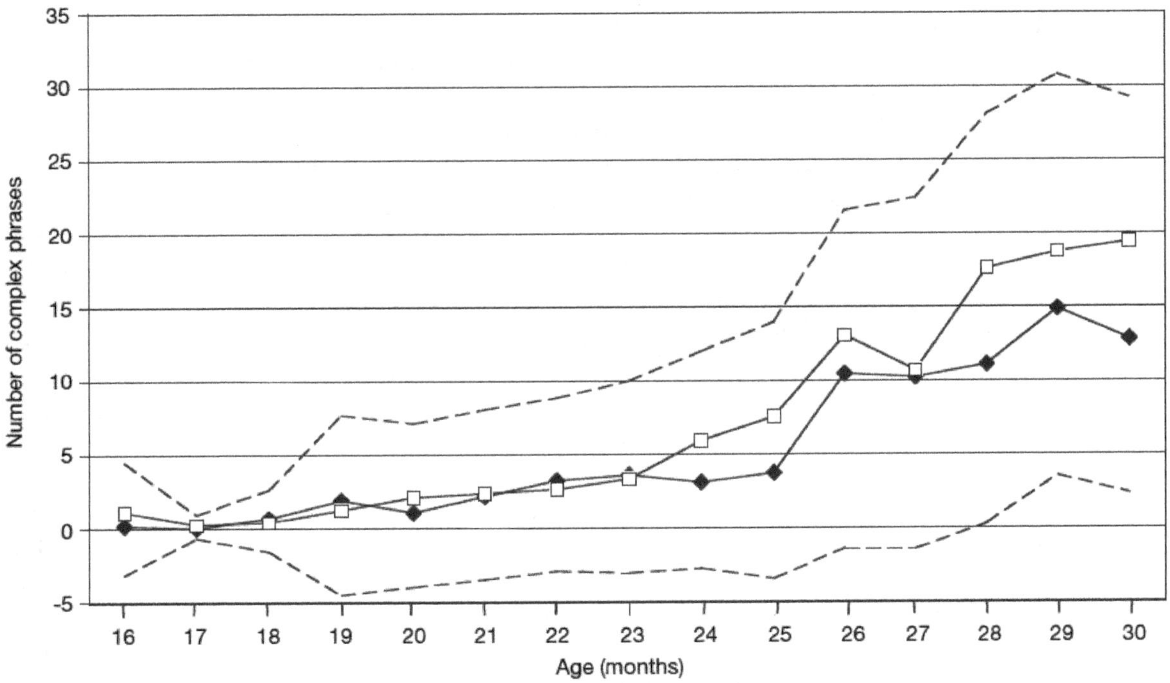

Figure 4.19. Mean *Complejidad de Frases* [Complexity] (Inventario II) scores by age and sex. (*Note:* The dashed lines represent ±1 standard deviation for the sexes combined.) (*Key:* —◆— boys; —□— girls.)

number of children at each age and education level. Multivariate analyses of variance (age level, education level) were conducted for three key Inventario I measures (*Comprensión de Palabras* [Words Understood], *Producción de Palabras* [Words Produced], and *Total de Gestos* [Total Gestures]), and three key Inventario II measures (*Producción de Palabras* [Words Produced], *M3L-Palabras* [M3L-*Words], and *Complejidad de Frases* [Complexity]). Modified Bonferroni tests were used to control Type I family-wise error rate for each of the simple comparisons at each age level. The alpha level was set at $p < .02$ for Inventario I and $p < .01$ for Inventario II for each of the simple effect t-tests that were performed.

Figure 4.20 presents the mean *Comprensión de las Primeras Frases* [Phrases Understood] scores as a function of age group and maternal education. Effects were evaluated using a 2 (age) × 3 (education) between-subjects analysis of variance. This analysis indicated significant main effects of age, $F(1, 757) = 301.0$, $p < .001$, and maternal education, $F(1, 757) = 3.5$, $p < .05$. The age × education interaction was not significant, $F(2, 757) = 1.9$, *ns*. Age accounted for 29% of the variance, whereas maternal education accounted for 1% of the variance. Examination of the simple effects applying Bonferroni corrections indicated that the mean scores for 8- to 12-month-old children whose mothers had the least education (no high school; $M = 15.4$, $SD = 7.1$) were significantly higher than those of the children whose mothers had some college ($M = 13.0$, $SD = 6.3$, $t(237) = 3.8$, $p < .01$). Mean vocabulary comprehension scores did not differ based on maternal education at the older ages ($M = 22.0$, $SD = 5.5$; $M = 22.4$, $SD = 5.2$; and $M = 21.7$, $SD = 5.6$ for the no high school, some high school, and some college groups, respectively).

Figure 4.21 presents the mean *Comprensión de Palabras* [Words Understood] scores at each age for each level of education. Effects were evaluated using a 2 (age group) × 3 (education) between-subjects analysis of variance. This analysis revealed a main effect of age, $F(1, 757) = 206.5$, $p < .05$, and a significant interaction between age and education, $F(2, 757) = 3.7$, $p < .05$. The main effect of maternal education was not significant, $F(2, 757) = 2.1$, *ns*. Age accounted for 21% of the variance, and the interaction accounted for 1% of the variance. Simple effect *t*-tests with Bonferroni corrections showed that at 8–12 months of age, children whose mothers had the least education (no high school; $M = 96.7$, $SD = 79.2$) had significantly higher reported comprehension vocabularies than children whose mothers had some college ($M = 63.3$, $SD = 55.6$), $t(237) = 3.8$, $p < .01$). Mean vocabulary comprehension scores did not differ as a function of maternal education at the older ages ($M = 161.8$, $SD = 97.3$; $M = 173.6$, $SD = 96.3$; and $M = 165.4$, $SD = 98.0$ for the no high school, some high school, and some college groups, respectively).

These findings closely parallel the results of the English CDI norming study, in which significantly higher scores for vocabulary comprehension were reported for children of mothers with lower education than for children of

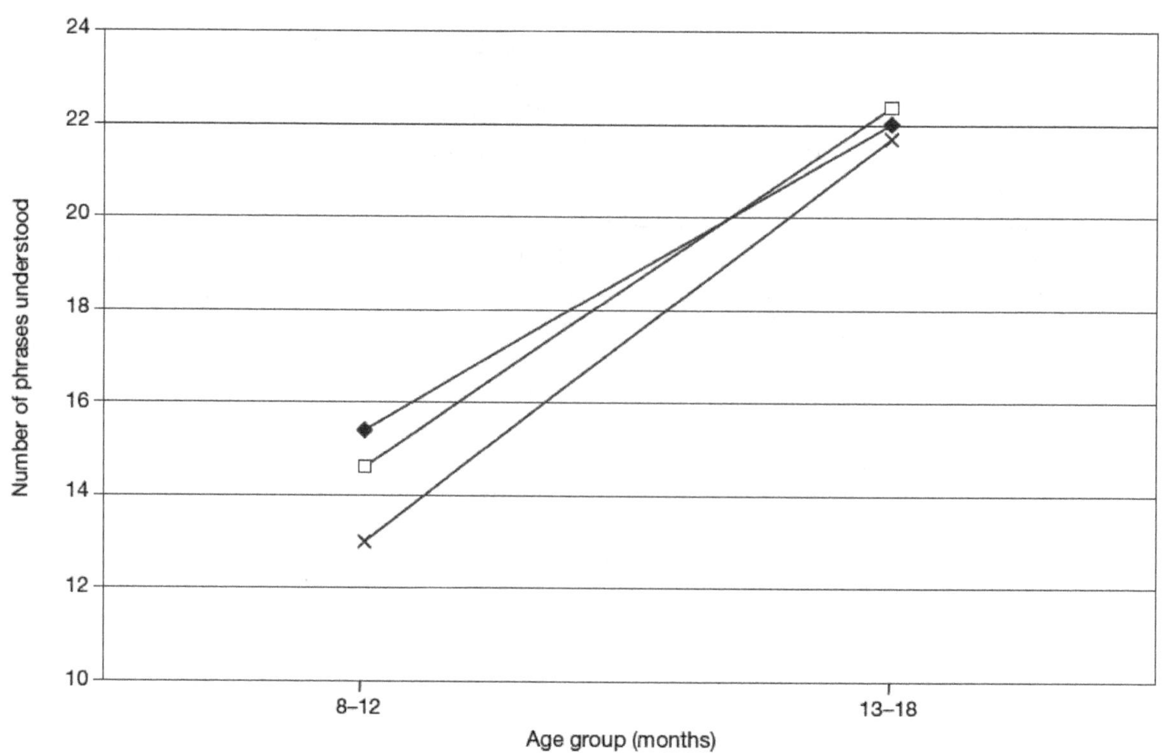

Figure 4.20. Mean *Comprensión de las Primeras Frases* [Phrases Understood] (Inventario I) scores by age group and education level. (*Key:* —◆— no high school; —□— some high school; —✕— some college.)

mothers with higher education (Fenson et al., 1992/1993). This finding is also consistent with an earlier report by Reznick (1990), in which he noted that parents with lower education gave higher estimates of vocabulary comprehension for their 12-month-old sons than parents with higher educational backgrounds. More recently, Feldman et al. (2000) reported an inverse relation between education level and scores on three measures from the English CDI: Words and Gestures (Comprehension of Phrases, Vocabulary Comprehension, and Vocabulary Production). These effects were also limited to the 8- to 12-month age range. Because of these findings, the word comprehension measure for children below 1 year of age should be treated with caution, particularly with children from families with lower education levels.

The mean *Producción de Palabras* [Words Produced] scores on Inventario I for each education level are shown in Figure 4.22. A 2 (age) × 3 (education) between-subjects analysis of variance for vocabulary production revealed a significant main effect of age, $F(1, 757) = 79.6, p < .01$], no main effect of maternal education, $F(2, 757) = 0.9$, *ns*, and no interaction $F(2, 757) = .35$, *ns*. Age accounted for 9.5% of the variance.

The mean *Total de Gestos* [Total Gestures] scores as a function of education and age level is shown in Figure 4.23. Results of a 2 (age) × 3 (education level) between-subjects analysis of variance indicated only a significant main effect of age, $F(1, 757) = 427.4, p < .01$]. There was no main effect of maternal

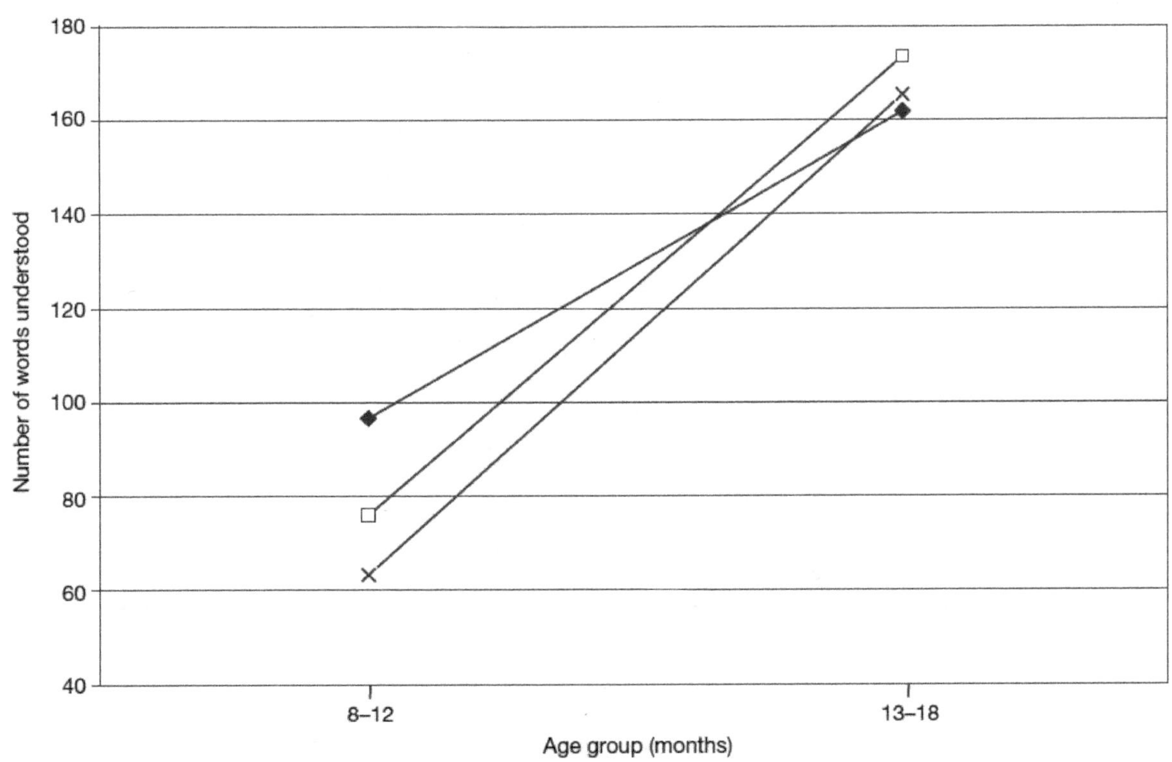

Figure 4.21. Mean *Comprensión de Palabras* [Words Understood] (Inventario I) scores by age group and education level. (*Key:* —◆— no high school; —□— some high school; —✕— some college.)

education level, $F(2, 757) = 0.2$, *ns*, and no significant interaction, $F(2, 757) = 1.7$, *ns*. Age accounted for 36% of the variance.

Figure 4.24 presents the mean *Producción de Palabras* [Words Produced] scores on Inventario II as a function of age and educational level. Results of a 3 (age) × 3 (education) between-subjects analysis of variance revealed a significant main effect of age, $F(2, 1{,}059) = 230.3$, $p < .001$, a significant main effect of maternal education, $F(2, 1{,}059) = 3.6$, $p < .05$, and a significant age by education interaction, $F(4, 1{,}059) = 4.6$, $p < .001$. Age accounted for 30% of the variance, maternal education accounted for 1% of the variance, and the interaction accounted for 2% of the variance. Post hoc comparisons at each of the three levels of age with modified Bonferroni corrections indicated that at 26–30 months of age, mothers in the most educated group reported that their children produced a significantly higher number of words on average ($M = 408.8$, $SD = 183.3$) than either the mothers with some high school ($M = 354.3$, $SD = 163.3$) or those with no high school ($M = 321.6$, $SD = 175.7$) ($p < .05$). Post hoc comparisons at the other two ages were not significant.

Mean scores for *M3L-Palabras* [M3L-*Words] at each education level are shown in Figure 4.25. Results of a 3 (age) × 3 (education) between-subjects analysis of variance revealed a significant main effect of age, $F(2, 1{,}033) = 214.0$, $p < .001$, a significant main effect of education, $F(2, 1{,}033) = 11.7$, $p < .001$, and a significant age by education interaction, $F(4, 1{,}033) = 7.7$, $p < .001$. Age

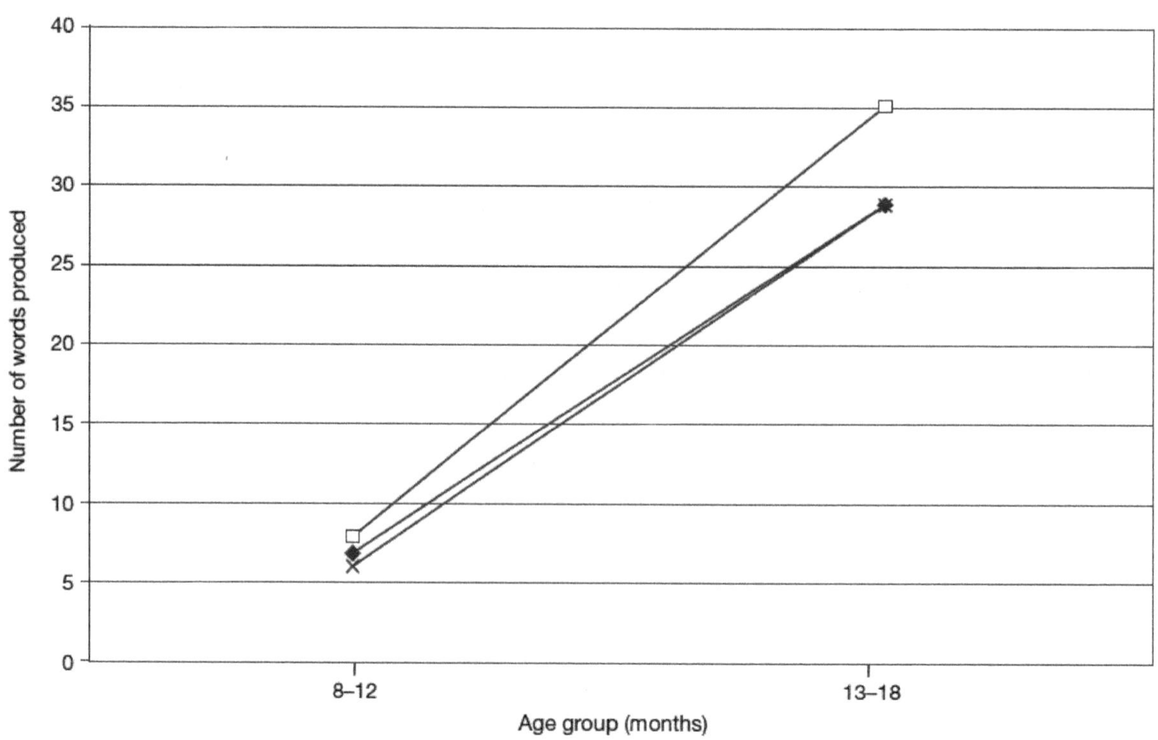

Figure 4.22. Mean *Producción de Palabras* [Words Produced] (Inventario I) scores by age group and education level. (*Key:* —◆— no high school; —□— some high school; —✕— some college.)

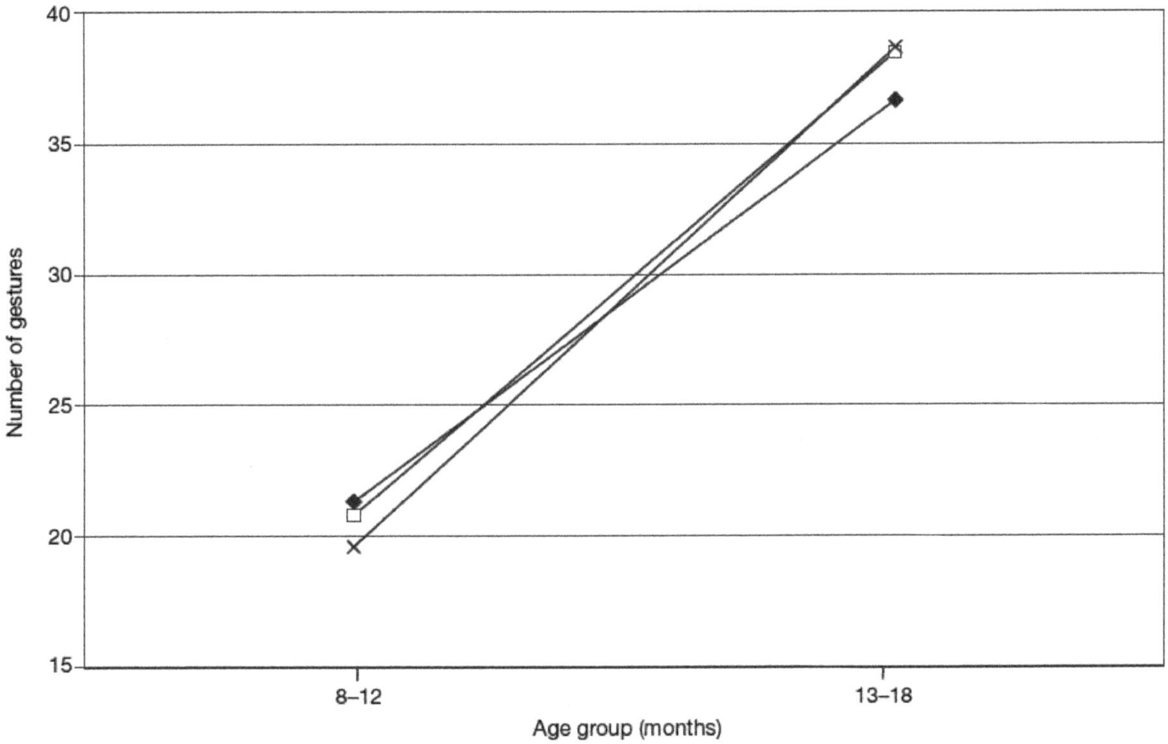

Figure 4.23. Mean *Total de Gestos* [Total Gestures] (Inventario I) scores by age group and education level. (*Key:* —◆— no high school; —□— some high school; —✕— some college.)

accounted for 29% of the variance, education level accounted for 2% of the variance, and the interaction accounted for 3% of the variance. Post hoc comparisons further indicated no significant differences based on the levels of maternal education at the two earliest ages (16–20 months and 21–25 months). A significant group difference, however, was found at 26–30 months of age. The mean score for the highest education group ($M = 5.4$, $SD = 2.7$) was significantly higher than that for either the no high school ($M = 3.8$, $SD = 2.4$) or some high school groups ($M = 4.1$, $SD = 1.8$), $p < .01$.

Figure 4.26 illustrates the differences in *Complejidad de Frases* [Complexity] by age and educational level. A 3 (age) × 3 (education) between-subjects analysis of variance revealed a significant main effect of age, $F(2, 1{,}059) = 192.3$, $p < .001$, a significant main effect of maternal education, $F(2, 1{,}059) = 7.8, p < .001$], and a significant age by education interaction, $F(4, 1{,}059) = 5.3$, $p < .001$]. Age accounted for 27% of the variance, education level accounted for 2% of the variance, and the interaction accounted for 2% of the variance. As was the case for *M3L-Palabras* [M3L-*Words], no significant differences in complexity scores were found for children with mothers with different levels of education at either 16–20 or 21–25 months. At 26–30 months, however, post hoc analyses applying a Bonferroni correction indicated that mean *Complejidad de Frases* [Complexity] scores were significantly higher for children whose mothers were the

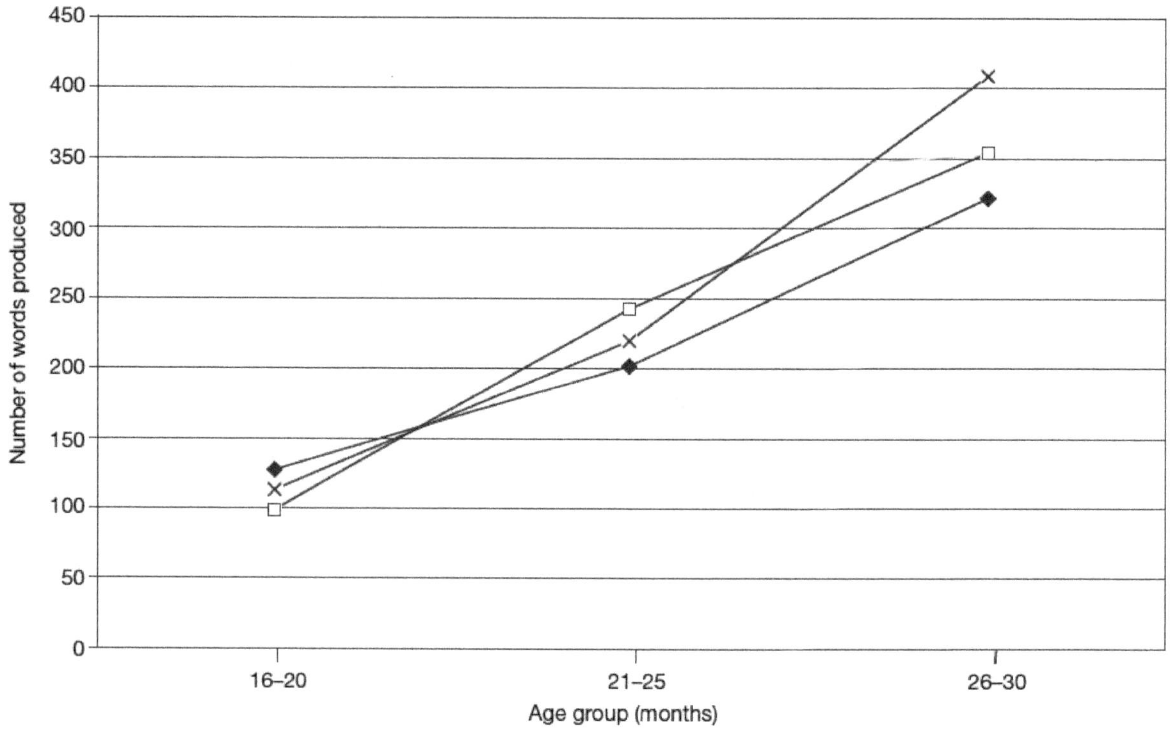

Figure 4.24. Mean *Producción de Palabras* [Words Produced] (Inventario II) by age group and education level. (*Key:* —◆— no high school; —□— some high school; —✕— some college.)

most educated (M = 17.9, SD = 14.4) compared with children whose mothers had lower levels of education (no high school: M = 11.2, SD = 12.4; some high school: M =13.1, SD = 12.2), $p < .05$.

In summary, the analyses of the impact of educational level are consistent with previous studies. For younger children in the age range of Inventario I, reported comprehension measures (*Comprensión de las Primeras Frases* [Phrases Understood] and *Comprensión de Palabras* [Words Understood]) are higher in children whose mothers have fewer years of education. An opposite pattern is seen for vocabulary and grammar production in reports of older children's language abilities. In the latter cases, reported scores of vocabulary and grammar are higher for children with more highly educated mothers than are those for children whose mothers have fewer years of education. More systematic analyses of the relationship between educational level and the assessment of language outcome with parent report are necessary to more fully understand the implications of these findings.

Birth Order

To evaluate birth order effects on communicative development, the means of first-born children were compared with those of later-born children (second or later) for the seven measures (i.e., *Comprensión de las Primeras Frases* [Phrases

Understood], *Comprensión de Palabras* [Words Understood], *Producción de Palabras* [Words Produced], and *Total de Gestos* [Total Gestures] on Inventario I; *Producción de Palabras* [Words Produced], *M3L-Palabras* [M3L-*Words], and *Complejidad de Frases* [Complexity] on Inventario II) using independent sample *t*-tests.

With respect to Inventario I, Table 4.27 presents the means and standard deviations for first- and later-born children for four key variables. In all cases, independent sample *t*-tests indicated that mean scores for first-born children were not significantly different from those for later-born children ($p > .05$). Thus, little evidence was found to support an influence of birth order on the acquisition of language milestones as assessed on Inventario I.

Table 4.28 presents the means and standard deviations as a function of birth order for three variables from Inventario II. In contrast to Inventario I findings, independent sample *t*-tests indicated significant differences between first- and later-born children for *Producción de Palabras* [Words Produced], $t(1{,}048) = 2.6, p < .01$, *M3L-Palabras* [M3L-*Words], $t(1{,}023) = 2.8, p < .005$, and *Complejidad de Frases* [Complexity], $t(1{,}048) = 2.3, p < .03$. These results indicate that for these lexical and grammatical measures, first-born children were likely to be more advanced, on average, than later-born children. Further correlational analyses indicated that although these effects are statistically significant, the contribution of birth order should only be characterized as minimal ($r = -.07$ to $-.09$). These findings are consistent with the significant but rela-

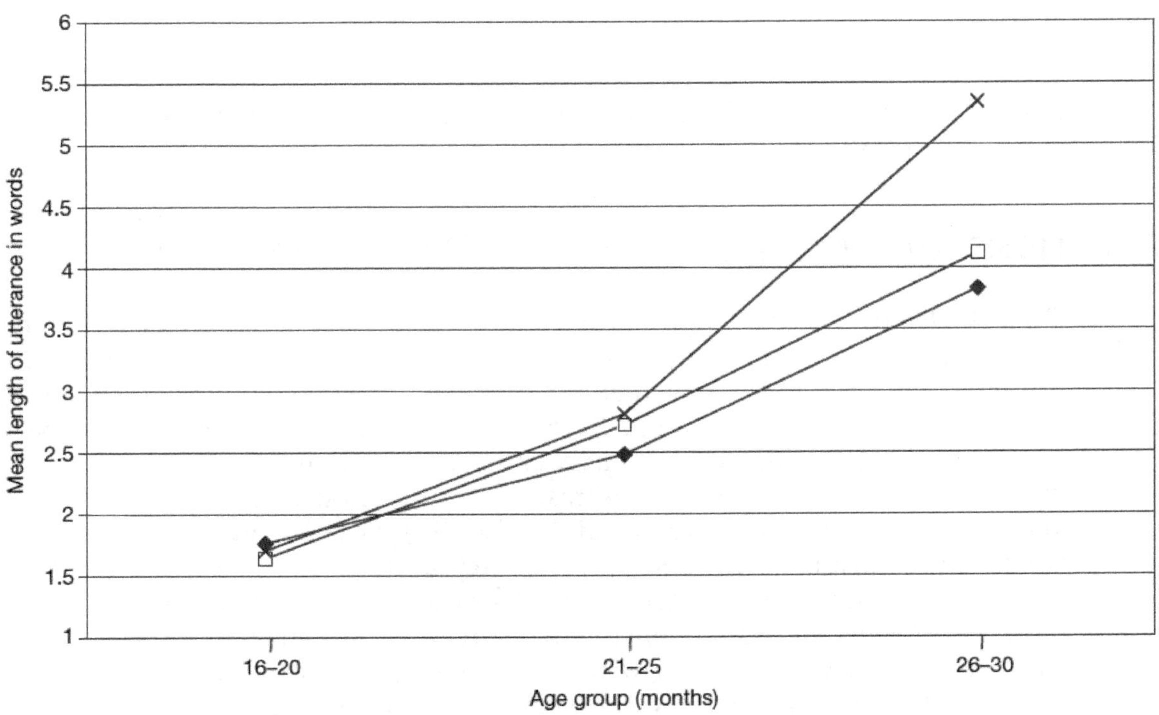

Figure 4.25. Mean *M3L-Palabras* [M3L-*Words] (Inventario II) scores by age group and education level. (*Key:* —◆— no high school; —□— some high school; —✕— some college.)

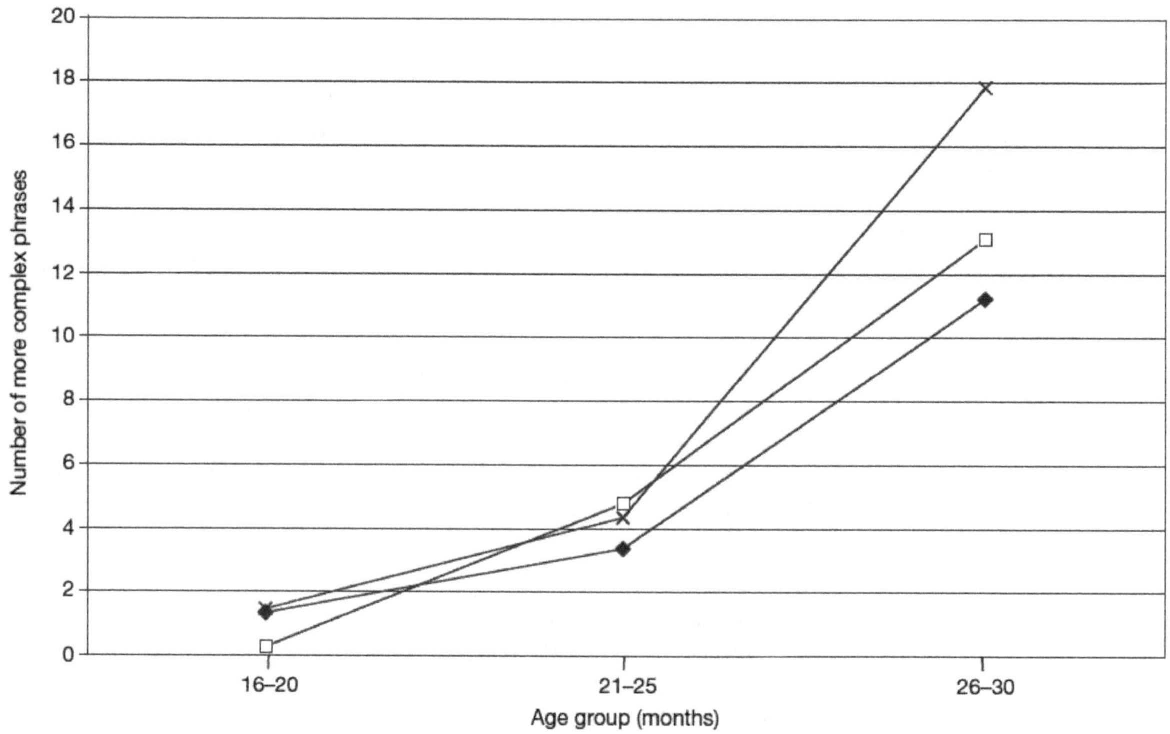

Figure 4.26. Mean *Complejidad de Frases* [Complexity] (Inventario II) scores by age group and education level. (*Key:* —◆— no high school; —□— some high school; —✕— some college.)

tively negligible correlations reported for the norming data of the English CDI (r = –.13 to –.05).

RELATIONS AMONG THE SUBSCALES OF THE INVENTARIOS

Table 4.29 shows the intercorrelations among the major components of Inventario I. Consistent with the findings from the norming of the English CDI (Fenson et al., 1992/1993), all of the major sections of the Inventario are significantly intercorrelated. However, some differences in degree of relationship are apparent. For example, gestures are strongly associated with the two comprehension measures (both single words and phrases) but only moderately correlated with vocabulary production. Bates et al. (1989), Tamis-LeMonda and Bornstein (1990), and Thal and Bates (1988) have also reported similar patterns. This finding is also consistent with those reported for the English CDI norms. As would be expected, the two comprehension measures are more highly correlated with each other than either one is with vocabulary production. The correlation, however, between vocabulary comprehension and production is moderate, whereas that between phrases understood and vocabulary production is considerably lower.

Table 4.27. Means and standard deviations for key Inventario I variables by birth order

	First-born (n = 334)		Later-born (n = 420)	
Inventario I variable	Mean	Standard deviation	Mean	Standard deviation
Comprensión de las Primeras Frases [Phrases Understood]	18.3	7.2	18.5	7.3
Comprensión de Palabras [Words Understood]	122.6	91.9	125.1	95.8
Producción de Palabras [Words Produced]	21.3	42.9	17.2	31.5
Total de Gestos [Total Gestures]	29.2	14.2	30.4	14.7

Table 4.28. Means and standards deviations for key Inventario II variables by birth order

	First-born (n = 504)		Later-born (n = 546)	
Inventario II variable	Mean	Standard deviation	Mean	Standard deviation
Producción de Palabras [Words Produced]	248.0	193.2	218.5	176.4
M3L-Palabras [M3L-*Words]	3.2	2.4	2.8	1.9
Complejidad de Frases [Complexity]	7.3	11.8	5.8	10.0

Table 4.29. Intercorrelations among the major components of Inventario I

Inventario I component	*Comprensión de Palabras* [Words Understood]	*Producción de Palabras* [Words Produced]	*Total de Gestos* [Total Gestures]
Comprensión de las Primeras Frases [Phrases Understood]	.67/.52	.30/.11	.67/.45
Comprensión de Palabras [Words Understood]		.53/.41	.73/.57
Producción de Palabras [Words Produced]			.47/.31

Note: $p < .01$ or better for all values in this table. The second value in each pair is the correlation with the effects of age partialled out.

Table 4.30. Intercorrelations among the major components of Inventario II

Inventario II component	*M3L-Palabras* [M3L-*Words]	*Complejidad de Frases* [Complexity]
Producción de Palabras [Words Produced]	.70/.55	.75/.67
M3L-Palabras [M3L-*Words]		.77/.67

Note: $p < .01$ or better for all values in this table. The second value in each pair is the correlation with the effects of age partialled out.

Table 4.30 shows the interrelations among the major components of Inventario II. All of these intercorrelations are statistically significant. These data indicate that vocabulary production is strongly correlated with each of the two grammar measures, and that the two grammatical measures are strongly associated with each other. Once again, these results parallel those found in the English language norming study (Fenson et al., 1992/1993).

RELIABILITY OF THE INVENTARIOS

Reliability refers to the consistency with which the items on a test or scale yield comparable indices of the abilities being assessed. There are two main types of reliability: internal consistency and test–retest reliability (see Sattler, 1988).

Internal Consistency

Internal consistency refers to the extent to which different items within the same category measure the same skills. Internal consistency was evaluated using Cronbach's coefficient alpha (α), a measure that is based on the split-half correlations across all possible item splits. For *Comprensión de Palabras* [Words Understood] and *Producción de Palabras* [Words Produced] on Inventario I and *Producción de Palabras* [Words Produced] on Inventario II, scores for each semantic category were treated as individual items (Inventario I: 22 semantic categories; Inventario II: 23 semantic categories). These indices demonstrated high internal consistency, producing alpha values of .94, .94, and .95, respectively. This is comparable to alphas of .95, .96, and .96 for the comprehension and production scales that were reported for the English CDIs (Fenson et al., 1992/1993).

For *Total de Gestos* [Total Gestures], each of the five gesture categories was treated as an individual item to compute Cronbach's alpha. The internal consistency for gestures was in the same range as the vocabulary measures (α = .89), comparable to internal consistency for gestures (α = .88) on the English CDI: Words and Gestures.

Cronbach's alpha was computed for *Complejidad de Frases* [Complexity], with each of the 37 items treated as an individual item. As with the other measures on the English CDIs and on the Inventarios, this scale demonstrated a high degree of internal consistency, producing an alpha of .98.

Test–Retest Reliability

Another type of reliability, termed test–retest reliability, measures the extent to which scores remain stable across two or more test sessions. Given the rapidity with which language skills can change over short periods of time and the uneven rates of language development among children, one would not expect the rank order for a group of children to remain constant for an extended period of time. At the same time, a considerable degree of stability would certainly be expected over a period of 6 weeks or less. Test–retest reliabilities were evaluated with families who participated in the pilot study using the penultimate version of the Inventarios (see Jackson-Maldonado et al., 1993). After completing one Inventario, a second Inventario was completed within 1 month ($n = 16$ for Inventario I; $n = 20$ for Inventario II).

For Inventario I, correlations from Time 1 to Time 2 were .97 ($p < .001$) for *Comprensión de Palabras* [Words Understood] and .81 ($p < .001$) for *Producción de Palabras* [Words Produced]. Partial correlations (with age removed) were $r = .66$ ($p < .001$) for *Comprensión de Palabras* [Words Understood] and .53 ($p < .01$) for *Producción de Palabras* [Words Produced]. For Inventario II, the full correlation for *Producción de Palabras* [Words Produced] was .70 ($p < .001$) from Time 1 to Time 2, and the partial correlation with age removed was .62 ($p < .01$). We should note that all of the parents in this earlier study had at least some high school education and completed the Inventario using the mail-in procedure (Jackson-Maldonado et al., 1993). These correlations provide evidence of excellent levels of reliability that are comparable to that reported for the English CDIs (see Jackson-Maldonado et al., 1993 for a full description of the findings regarding test–retest reliability of the Inventarios).

VALIDITY OF THE INVENTARIOS

Face Validity

A test is said to have face validity if it appears to measure the targeted domain. Face validity is very important for gaining and maintaining a concerted effort by the parent when completing an Inventario. The professional appearance of the Inventarios encourages the parent to take the form seriously. Parents will probably be more influenced, however, by the structure and content of the forms. Most parents will want to provide a detailed and full account of their child's communicative skills. The parent will notice that each of the Inventarios samples a wide range of communicative skills in considerable depth. That impression should, in turn, increase the probability that the parent will regard the inventory as presenting an opportunity to portray his or her child's developing skills accurately and completely.

Content Validity

Another important type of validity is content validity, defined as the extent to which the content of the scale maps onto the content that the investigator hopes to assess. Content validity is determined by examining the features of an instrument to determine whether the components relate to the skills that the instrument is designed to measure. The case for content validity of the Inventarios rests on the assertion that the two forms sample the major features of communicative development across the 8- to 30-month age range. The items within each subscale were drawn from published Spanish language diary studies, doctoral dissertation databases, unpublished Spanish language data, comparable items on Spanish language tests, and comments made by parents when consulted about the penultimate version of the instrument. Based on developmental research, Inventario I covers major domains of early communication, including language comprehension, vocabulary production, and use of gestures, whereas Inventario II focuses on vocabulary production and the production of a range of grammatical forms.

Convergent Validity

Additional evidence of validity rests on the fact that the developmental functions obtained with the various subscales correspond closely to the developmental functions that have been reported for the same variables in observational studies. We regard the close parallels between data obtained with the Inventarios and developmental patterns reported in the literature as extremely important evidence of convergent validity. Although the parallels between the growth curves derived from the Inventarios and patterns reported in the literature do not quite fit the traditional meaning of convergent validity (Anastasi, 1988), the term fits better than do other terms.

The developmental functions are monotonic, the "floor" for each measure corresponds closely to the age of onset reported in the literature, and rates of development correspond to longitudinal and cross-sectional findings reported in studies using other techniques. With a few exceptions, the range of variation observed around each function also appears to be quite credible, based on what is known from observational studies. A single exception is the variation in word comprehension observed at 8 months of age, when some of the parents reported receptive vocabularies that were much higher than estimates in prior studies. This phenomenon was also seen in the English sample, and we suspect that some parents have applied a different and more liberal criterion than we had in mind in both cases. It is also possible, of course, that the other methods underestimate vocabulary comprehension. Overall, however, there appears to be an excellent match between our intent and the parents' interpretations.

Although the English version of the grammatical scales showed impressive convergent validity, there was no guarantee that similar scales would perform as well in a highly inflected and morphologically complex language like Spanish. Also, the English and Spanish scales are not alternate versions of the same thing: they are separate measures. These facts make the strong evidence found for validity quite impressive. The developmental functions obtained for the grammar scales correspond closely to reports in the literature. This includes the relative time of onset for production of word combinations and the acceleration in grammatical complexity observed between 18 months (when grammatical inflections began to appear in the norming sample) and 30 months (when most children in the sample used a variety of grammatical inflections and function words). Literature has shown that verb morphology, including tense, aspect, and person, begins to appear as early as 20 months (Aguado Alonso, 1989; Anderson, 1995; Beléndez-Soltero, 1980; Dato, 1975; Fernández Martínez, 1994; Gathercole et al., 1999; González, 1983; Hernández Pina, 1984; Jackson-Maldonado & Maldonado, 2001; Maez, 1983; Merino & Spencer, 1983) and that early phrases are extended to include function words and subordinate phrases. Because we can assume that very few parents have "textbook" knowledge of child language, we conclude that the developmental functions obtained with the Inventarios correspond to reports in the literature because parents and psycholinguists are listening to and reporting the same developmental phenomena.

Nevertheless, it is important to determine whether the scores obtained for individual children with the Inventarios correspond to scores the same children might obtain in laboratory testing and/or home observations. This brings us to correlational studies of the concurrent and predictive validity of the Inventarios and their predecessors.

Concurrent Validity

Concurrent validity was determined by assessing the relation between parent report (i.e., Inventario scores) and child performance on associated laboratory measures.

Inventario I The validation of Inventario I is difficult to document because there are very few reliable and valid behavioral measures of language and gesture for children in this age range. Evidence must come from comparison with measures of spontaneous communication and play. In a study of nineteen 10-month-old and twenty 12-month-old children living in Mexico (Jackson-Maldonado, 1994), measures of language and gesture use in naturalistic communication samples were compared with responses on Inventario I. Only 37% of the 10-month-olds produced more than two communicative acts. Thus, there was insufficient data in the communication sample to use for comparison with the Inventario. Seventy five percent of the 12-month-olds produced more than two communicative acts, providing sufficient data for analysis. The correlation between *Producción de Palabras* [Words Produced] on Inventario I and number of different words produced in a spontaneous communication sample was moderately strong ($r = .61$, $p < .005$). These data indicate good reliability for 12-month-old children on this measure. The correlation between *Total de Gestos* [Total Gestures] and the number of different conventionalized communicative gestures (e.g., shaking the head "no," shrugging the shoulders for "All gone") used in the spontaneous communication sample was also moderate ($r = .47$, $p < .04$). When *Gestos Tempranos* [Early Gestures] and *Gestos Tardíos* [Later Gestures] were evaluated separately, the data indicated that the overall relationship is accounted for by *Gestos Tardíos* [Later Gestures]. *Gestos Tardíos* [Later Gestures] is significantly correlated with conventionalized gesture use in the laboratory ($r = .50$, $p < .02$), whereas scores on *Gestos Tempra-*

nos [Early Gestures] are not. This suggests reasonable validity for the gesture section of Inventario I and suggests that further research to examine more specific gestures may be worthwhile.

Inventario II Thal, Jackson-Maldonado, and Acosta (2000) compared *Producción de Palabras* [Words Produced] on Inventario II and laboratory measures of word production in 39 typically developing, healthy children living in Querétaro and Mexico City, Mexico. Twenty of the children were 20 months old, and nineteen were 28 months old. All came from middle- to upper middle-class families as determined by parental occupation and education. Two behavioral measures of language production (which were part of a larger study of the relation between language and nonlinguistic cognition) were used. One was an object-naming task (adapted from Bates et al., 1989, and Thal & Bates, 1988) in which 10 real objects were presented to the child, one at a time. The child was allowed to play with each object for 30 seconds, during which time he or she usually named it. If the child didn't name the object, the experimenter asked "*¿Qué es eso?*" ["What is this?"] and waited for a response. The names for the objects (*sombrero* [hat], *carro* [car], *peine* [comb], *cuchara* [spoon], *flor* [flower], *taza* [cup], *avión* [airplane], *muñeca* [baby doll], *perro* [dog], and *teléfono* [telephone]) all appear on the *Lista de Vocabulario* [Vocabulary Checklist] of Inventario II. An additional language measure (number of different words produced) was derived from a 35-minute spontaneous language sample.

For the 20-month-old children, the correlation was .69 ($p < .01$) between *Producción de Palabras* [Words Produced] and the naming task and .66 ($p < .05$) for *Producción de Palabras* [Words Produced] and the number of different words in the spontaneous language sample. This moderately high correlation is higher than that reported by Dale et al. (1989) for typically developing English-speaking 20-month-olds on a similar measure of vocabulary. Dale reported a correlation of .54 between CDI vocabulary and number of items correct on an expressive language subscale of the Bayley Scales of Infant Development (Bayley, 1969, 1993). Furthermore, Bates et al. (1988) reported a high correlation using a very early version of the CDI and a lexical index derived from 2 to 3 hours of spontaneous language at 20 months of age ($r = .83$). The correlation reported by Bates et al. is considerably higher than that reported by either Dale et al. (1989) or Thal et al. (2000). There are several possible sources of the discrepancy. First, Bates et al. (1988) used a longitudinal cohort, collected the parent report information via direct interview, and sampled language in the children's home and in the laboratory. Second, that longitudinal study was a substantially richer sample than the cross-sectional study by Thal et al. In the Thal et al. study, parents filled out the inventory and returned it without being directly interviewed, samples were obtained in only one setting, and only 30 minutes of spontaneous language were used. Third, Dale et al. (1989) only measured vocabulary. Given these substantial methodological differences, the similarity between the results is noteworthy. Taken together, there is considerable evidence that Inventario II is a valid measure of vocabulary in Spanish-speaking toddlers at 20 months of age.

For 28-month-old children, the number of reported *Producción de Palabras* [Words Produced] was correlated moderately highly with object naming ($r = .68$) and moderately with the number of different words in the language sample ($r = .56$). These findings are somewhat lower than, but comparable to, the correlations between the CDI and behavioral measures of vocabulary reported by Dale (1991) for younger English-speaking children ($r = .73$ with the Expressive One-Word Picture Vocabulary Test [EOWPVT; Gardner, 1981] and $r = .74$ with number of different words produced in a language sample for 24-month-olds). These correlations are also in the same range as those reported for older preschoolers with language delays by Thal, O'Hanlon, et al. (1999) ($r = .86$ with the EOWPVT and $r = .78$ with number of different words in the language sample for 39- to 49-month-olds with specific language delay). In general, then, the correlations for the Spanish-speaking 28-month-olds are respectable and significant, indicating that Inventario II is a valid measure of vocabulary production at this age.

Thal et al. (2000) also examined the relationship between mean length of utterance in words from a language sample (M3L-Words) and the two measures of grammar on Inventario II, *M3L-Palabras* [M3L-*Words] and *Complejidad de Frases* [Complexity] in 28-month-olds. The correlation between the language sample M3L-Words and Inventario II *M3L-Palabras* [M3L-*Words] was .68, and the correlation between the language sample M3L-Words and *Complejidad de Frases* [Complexity] was .73. These values are comparable to the correlations reported by Dale (1991) for English-speaking 24-month-olds (CDI M3L × language sample M3L-Words, $r = .74$; CDI Complexity × language sample M3L-Words, $r = .76$). Similar results were reported by Thal, O'Hanlon, et al. (1999) for older children with specific language delay ($r = .68$ to $.69$). These results provide strong evidence for the validity of the Inventario measures of grammar for Spanish-speaking 28-month-olds and underscore the comparability of summary data from Spanish- and English-speaking parents.

Inventario II also contains a section, *Formas de Verbos* [*Verb Forms], in which parents are asked to indicate which *Presente* [*Present] (12 items), *Pasado* [*Past] (6 items), and *Imperativo* [*Imperative] (6 items) forms are used by their child. To test the validity of this section of Inventario II, Jackson-Maldonado (2000) examined the correlation between reported use of verbs and verb use during a spontaneous language sample of 35 middle-class Spanish-speaking children (20–28 months of age). The correlation between *Formas de Verbos* [*Verb Forms] (24 items total) and the number of different verbs that were conjugated during the language sample was .70 ($p < .0001$). When frequency of conjugated verb use was evaluated for each of the three subsections individually, the correlation between reported and spontaneous verb use was high for two of the sections, with $r = .62$ ($p < .0001$) for present-tense and .67 ($p < .0001$) for past-tense conjugations. The correlation for imperative forms, on the other hand, was very low (.03) and nonsignificant. Thus, there is ample support for the validity of the present- and past-tense verb conjugations on Inventario II. The validity of parent report of their child's use of the imperative form, however, was not demonstrated. Further study is required to explore valid means of assessing children's use of the imperative form.

Concurrent Validity in Bilingual Populations An advantage of having similar parent report instruments in English and Spanish is that the two instruments can be used concurrently with children who are exposed to both languages. In a study using the CDIs and Inventarios, Marchman and Martínez-Sussmann (2002) examined vocabulary development in children who heard both English and Spanish at least 12 hours per week ($n = 26$), typically from birth. Participants ranged in age from 23–34 months old ($M = 27.9$ months). All of the families lived in a large metropolitan area of the United States. Parents were generally proficient in both languages, and almost half of the families (42%) preferred to use both English and Spanish in the home. Children were exposed to different amounts of English and Spanish, ranging from 14% English (86% Spanish) to 3% Spanish (97% English). The families also participated in two laboratory play sessions, one in English and one in Spanish, conducted approximately 2 weeks apart. Each session used a different "home" play partner (e.g., mother, father) and "lab" play partner. All of the lab partners were proficient in both English and Spanish but only spoke to the child in the assigned "language of the day." During each lab session, children participated in an object-naming task (adapted from Thal et al., 2000) and in a free-play session during which 24 minutes of spontaneous language sample data were collected.

The results indicated strong correlations between parent report and laboratory measures of vocabulary production in both English and Spanish (CDI Vocabulary Production × English Naming, $r = .72$, $p < .001$; *Producción de Palabras* × Spanish Naming, $r = .78$, $p < .0001$). Similarly high correlations were observed between the parent report measures and number of different words (NDW) produced from the language sample (CDI Vocabulary Production × English NDW, $r = .79$, $p < .0001$; *Producción de Palabras* × Spanish NDW, $r = .60$, $p < .01$). In contrast, the cross-language correlations were low and nonsignificant (ranging from –.19 to .08). These data demonstrate concurrent validity levels for word production in these potentially bilingual children that were as high or higher than those observed in monolingual populations (see Fenson et al., 1992/1993, and Thal et al., 2000). Similarly strong correlations were also observed for the parent report measures of grammar compared with language sample measures (e.g., M3L-Words), ranging from .53 to .71. Clearly more studies are required to be fully confident of the validity of the CDIs and Inventarios when used with children with English and Spanish exposure. These data suggest, however, that the CDIs and Inventarios demonstrate good potential as valid tools for the assessment of early language development in toddlers who are learning both English and Spanish.

Predictive Validity

An instrument possesses predictive validity to the extent that components of the instrument measured at one point in time correlate with the same or other components of the instrument measured at subsequent points in time. Previous research with the English language version of the inventories has provided substantial evidence for the predictive power of parent report instruments across the first 3 years of life (Bates et al., 1979; Bates et al., 1988; Dale et al., 1989). For example, Bates et al. (1988) found correlations in the range of .60 to

.80 between estimates of productive vocabulary at 20 months (using parent report) and various measures of vocabulary and grammar at 28 months (using observational data).

Predictive validity of the vocabulary sections of the Inventarios was established with a study of the penultimate versions of the Inventarios (Jackson-Maldonado et al., 1993). Correlations ranged from .70 to .97 ($p < .001$), and partial correlations (with the effects of age removed) ranged from .53 to .66 ($p < .01$) for Inventarios administered 1 month apart. These data provide further evidence for the predictive validity of the Inventarios.

CONCLUSIONS

The MacArthur CDIs have been adapted to more than 20 different languages, attesting to the usefulness of parent report as a tool for language assessment in young children. The norming study of the Inventarios provides key foundational information regarding a culturally and linguistically appropriate parent report measure of the acquisition of Mexican Spanish.

The Inventarios will be very useful throughout Latin America, where Spanish is the first language. These instruments will also fill a growing need in the United States, where Spanish is the language spoken in an increasing number of family, school, and clinical settings. In Mexico, and in the Spanish-speaking world in general, few language assessment instruments are available, especially for the earliest stages of development. The Inventarios were normed on speakers of Mexican Spanish but could be used with speakers of other regional dialects of Spanish, so long as appropriate modifications are made (see Appendix C for some examples of dialectal variants). The Inventarios can help serve many goals in both research on language development and clinical assessment in that they provide reliable, valid, normed instruments for Spanish-speaking children (see also Thal et al., 2000). The Inventarios have the advantage of using the method of parent report, which has been shown to be a time-saving means of obtaining information about early language. They also have counterparts in many other languages, creating better opportunities for cross-linguistic research and research on bilingualism and the assessment of bilingual children. For Spanish and English, the computer-based CDI Scoring Program (see Chapter 2 for more information) provides monolingual scores and norms for either language and a composite score for children who are learning both Spanish and English (see Marchman & Martínez-Sussmann, 2002).

Although the Inventarios will be useful for many purposes, extreme caution must be applied when they are administered to children who have little or no representation in the norming sample. For example, children from Mexican families with very low income and education are not adequately represented. Further research is needed in order to determine whether the Inventarios are valid and reliable for children from these families.

Researchers or clinicians may wish to use the Inventarios with two other groups of children who are not represented in the norming sample: children growing up in a bilingual environment and children with language delay who are older than the norming sample. Studies by Conboy (2001), Conboy and Mills (2001), and Marchman and Martínez-Sussman (2002) have shown that the Inventarios provide valid assessment information about bilingual children. Because the Thal, O'Hanlon, et al. (1999) study showed that the English CDIs are valid for use with older children with language delays who speak English, one could reasonably presume that the Inventarios can be used successfully with older children with language delay who speak Spanish. Further research is necessary, however, to definitively demonstrate the Inventarios' validity with these children. We are currently collecting data from older Mexican children with language delay, Down syndrome, serious hearing impairment, and other disorders that have accompanying language delays in order to examine the reliability and validity of the Inventarios with these children.

Although the success of the Inventarios as a research and clinical tool has been demonstrated in a number of studies, it must also be acknowledged that several factors may affect the validity of the information provided by the instruments. Clearly, it is imperative that users of the Inventarios be informed about both the advantages and the limitations of the instruments, in particular cases and for particular purposes. In this manual, we have offered guidelines for appropriate administration and interpretation for a variety of purposes. Nevertheless, the ultimate success of this tool remains in the hands of the individual users who must be aware of and sensitive to the specific characteristics, concerns, and requirements of their target children and families.

5

PERCENTILE TABLES AND FIGURES FOR THE INVENTARIOS

These percentile tables and figures are fitted values derived from data collected for the norming of the Inventarios (Inventario I N = 778 [n = 373 girls, 405 boys]; Inventario II N = 1,094 [n = 541 girls, 553 boys]). See Chapter 2 for detailed instructions on scoring the Inventarios and creating *Informes del Niño/a* [Child Report Forms].

Table 5.1. Fitted percentile scores for *Comprensión de las Primeras Frases* [Phrases Understood] (Inventario I)—both sexes combined

%ile rank	Age in months										
	8	**9**	**10**	**11**	**12**	**13**	**14**	**15**	**16**	**17**	**18**
99	27	27	27	27	28	28	28	28	28	28	28
95	25	26	26	27	27	27	28	28	28	28	28
90	22	23	24	25	26	27	27	28	28	28	28
85	18	20	22	24	25	26	27	27	28	28	28
80	15	18	20	22	24	25	26	27	28	28	28
75	14	16	19	21	23	25	26	27	27	28	28
70	13	15	18	20	22	24	25	26	27	28	28
65	12	14	17	19	21	23	24	25	26	27	28
60	12	14	16	18	20	22	23	24	25	26	27
55	11	13	15	17	19	21	23	24	25	26	27
50	10	12	14	16	18	20	22	23	24	25	26
45	9	11	13	15	17	19	21	23	24	25	26
40	9	10	12	14	16	18	20	21	23	24	25
35	8	10	11	13	15	17	18	20	22	23	24
30	7	9	11	12	14	16	18	19	21	22	24
25	6	8	9	11	13	15	17	18	20	22	23
20	5	6	8	10	11	13	15	17	19	21	22
15	5	6	7	8	10	11	13	15	17	19	20
10	4	4	5	7	8	10	11	13	15	17	19
5	2	3	4	5	6	7	9	10	12	14	16

Table 5.2. Fitted percentile scores for *Comprensión de las Primeras Frases* [Phrases Understood] (Inventario I)—girls

%ile rank	Age in months										
	8	9	10	11	12	13	14	15	16	17	18
99	26	27	27	27	27	28	28	28	28	28	28
95	25	26	26	27	27	27	28	28	28	28	28
90	22	24	25	26	26	27	27	28	28	28	28
85	20	22	23	24	25	26	27	27	28	28	28
80	18	20	22	23	25	26	26	27	28	28	28
75	16	18	20	22	24	25	26	27	27	28	28
70	14	17	19	21	22	24	25	26	27	27	28
65	13	15	17	19	21	23	24	25	26	27	27
60	11	14	16	18	20	22	23	25	26	27	27
55	11	13	15	17	19	21	23	24	25	26	27
50	11	13	15	17	18	20	22	23	24	25	26
45	11	13	14	16	18	20	21	22	24	25	25
40	10	11	13	15	17	19	20	22	23	24	25
35	9	10	12	14	16	17	19	21	22	23	24
30	7	9	11	12	14	16	18	20	21	22	24
25	6	8	9	11	13	15	17	18	20	22	23
20	6	7	9	10	12	14	15	17	19	20	22
15	5	6	7	9	10	12	14	16	18	19	21
10	4	5	6	7	8	10	12	14	15	17	19
5	3	3	4	5	6	7	9	10	12	14	15

Table 5.3. Fitted percentile scores for *Comprensión de las Primeras Frases* [Phrases Understood] (Inventario I)—boys

%ile rank	Age in months										
	8	9	10	11	12	13	14	15	16	17	18
99	26	26	27	27	27	27	28	28	28	28	28
95	24	25	26	26	27	27	27	28	28	28	28
90	21	23	24	25	26	27	27	28	28	28	28
85	18	20	22	23	24	26	26	27	28	28	28
80	15	18	20	22	24	25	26	27	27	28	28
75	13	15	18	21	23	24	26	27	27	28	28
70	12	14	17	20	22	24	25	26	27	28	28
65	12	14	16	19	21	23	24	25	26	27	28
60	11	13	16	18	20	22	24	25	26	27	27
55	10	12	14	17	19	21	22	24	25	26	27
50	8	10	13	15	18	20	22	23	25	26	27
45	8	10	12	14	16	18	20	22	23	25	26
40	7	9	11	13	15	18	20	21	23	24	25
35	7	9	10	12	14	16	18	20	22	23	24
30	6	8	10	11	13	16	18	19	21	23	24
25	6	7	9	10	12	14	16	18	20	21	23
20	5	6	8	9	11	13	15	17	19	21	22
15	4	5	7	8	10	11	13	15	17	19	20
10	3	4	5	6	8	9	11	12	14	16	17
5	2	3	3	4	5	6	8	9	11	13	15

Table 5.4. Fitted percentile scores for *Comprensión de Palabras* [Words Understood] (Inventario I)—both sexes combined

%ile rank	Age in months										
	8	**9**	**10**	**11**	**12**	**13**	**14**	**15**	**16**	**17**	**18**
99	170	227	282	329	364	388	404	414	420	424	426
95	145	175	206	237	268	296	322	344	362	377	389
90	127	150	174	199	225	250	275	298	318	337	353
85	109	128	149	171	194	218	242	265	287	308	326
80	91	108	127	148	171	194	218	242	265	287	307
75	81	96	113	132	153	174	197	220	243	265	286
70	73	87	101	118	136	155	175	197	218	240	261
65	61	73	87	103	121	141	162	185	208	231	254
60	50	61	74	90	107	127	148	171	195	220	245
55	41	51	63	78	96	115	138	162	188	215	242
50	36	45	56	70	86	105	126	149	175	201	228
45	30	38	48	60	76	93	114	138	163	191	219
40	25	32	41	52	66	83	102	125	151	178	207
35	20	26	34	44	56	72	90	112	137	165	195
30	15	20	26	35	46	59	76	96	120	147	177
25	12	16	22	29	38	49	64	82	103	128	157
20	10	13	18	23	31	41	54	70	90	114	141
15	7	9	13	17	24	32	43	57	75	97	123
10	4	6	8	11	16	22	31	43	59	79	104
5	1	1	2	4	5	9	13	20	31	47	69

Table 5.5. Fitted percentile scores for *Comprensión de Palabras* [Words Understood] (Inventario I)—girls

%ile rank	Age in months										
	8	9	10	11	12	13	14	15	16	17	18
99	219	256	290	321	346	367	383	396	405	412	417
95	187	215	242	269	294	316	336	354	368	380	390
90	144	164	186	209	232	254	275	296	314	331	346
85	137	154	171	189	207	225	243	261	278	294	310
80	114	130	148	167	187	207	228	248	268	286	304
75	90	105	122	140	159	179	200	222	243	263	283
70	80	93	109	126	144	164	184	206	227	248	269
65	68	81	95	111	129	148	168	190	211	233	255
60	53	64	78	93	111	130	151	174	198	222	246
55	41	51	64	79	96	116	138	163	188	215	242
50	35	44	55	69	84	103	123	147	172	198	225
45	31	39	49	61	75	92	111	132	156	182	208
40	29	36	45	55	67	82	99	118	139	162	186
35	25	31	39	48	59	71	87	104	123	145	168
30	21	26	32	40	50	61	75	91	109	130	152
25	17	22	27	35	44	55	68	84	102	123	147
20	11	14	19	26	34	44	58	75	95	119	146
15	9	12	16	20	27	34	44	57	72	91	112
10	4	6	8	12	16	23	31	43	58	77	101
5	1	2	2	3	5	8	12	17	26	37	54

Table 5.6. Fitted percentile scores for *Comprensión de Palabras* [Words Understood] (Inventario I)—boys

%ile rank	Age in months										
	8	9	10	11	12	13	14	15	16	17	18
99	106	156	215	273	324	362	388	404	415	421	424
95	101	140	185	232	278	319	351	376	393	405	414
90	112	136	162	191	220	249	277	302	325	345	362
85	91	112	136	162	190	219	247	275	300	323	343
80	82	99	119	141	165	190	216	242	268	291	313
75	78	93	109	128	148	169	192	215	238	260	282
70	66	79	94	111	130	150	172	195	218	241	263
65	53	65	79	95	113	133	156	179	204	229	254
60	44	55	68	84	102	123	146	171	197	224	250
55	37	46	58	73	90	110	132	157	184	212	240
50	32	41	52	66	83	102	125	151	179	208	237
45	27	35	45	57	72	91	112	137	164	193	223
40	21	28	37	48	63	81	102	127	155	186	218
35	16	21	29	39	52	68	89	114	142	174	208
30	13	18	24	33	44	59	77	99	126	156	189
25	11	15	20	27	36	49	65	84	108	137	168
20	7	10	14	20	27	37	50	66	87	112	142
15	5	7	10	14	20	28	39	54	74	99	129
10	3	4	6	9	13	18	26	36	50	68	92
5	1	1	2	3	5	8	12	19	29	43	64

Table 5.7. Fitted percentile scores for *Producción de Palabras* [Words Produced] (Inventario I)—both sexes combined

%ile rank	Age in months										
	8	**9**	**10**	**11**	**12**	**13**	**14**	**15**	**16**	**17**	**18**
99	30	42	59	80	106	138	175	214	253	289	321
95	14	20	27	38	51	69	91	118	150	185	222
90	7	10	15	21	29	41	56	77	102	132	167
85	5	8	11	15	21	28	39	53	70	93	120
80	5	6	9	12	16	22	29	39	52	68	89
75	4	5	7	9	12	16	21	28	37	48	62
70	3	4	5	7	10	13	18	24	32	42	56
65	2	3	4	6	8	10	14	19	25	40	55
60	2	2	3	5	6	9	12	16	21	39	54
55	2	2	3	4	6	8	10	14	19	33	53
50	0	0	1	1	2	4	7	11	19	31	51
45	0	0	1	1	2	3	6	10	16	27	44
40	0	0	0	0	1	2	4	8	15	26	43
35	0	0	0	0	1	2	3	6	12	24	41
30	0	0	0	0	0	1	1	3	8	20	40
25	0	0	0	0	0	0	1	3	6	15	33
20	0	0	0	0	0	0	1	2	5	11	24
15	0	0	0	0	0	0	0	1	2	5	11
10	0	0	0	0	0	0	0	0	0	1	2
5	0	0	0	0	0	0	0	0	0	0	0

Table 5.8. Fitted percentile scores for *Producción de Palabras* [Words Produced] (Inventario I)—girls

%ile rank	Age in months										
	8	9	10	11	12	13	14	15	16	17	18
99	26	34	45	58	74	94	117	143	172	203	234
95	17	23	32	43	57	76	99	126	158	192	227
90	9	13	18	25	35	49	67	91	119	153	191
85	6	8	12	17	24	35	49	68	92	123	158
80	5	7	10	13	18	25	34	46	62	82	106
75	5	6	8	11	15	19	25	33	43	56	72
70	4	5	7	9	12	16	21	28	36	48	62
65	3	4	5	7	9	13	17	23	31	41	60
60	2	3	4	6	8	11	14	20	27	39	58
55	2	2	3	5	6	9	12	17	24	38	58
50	0	1	1	2	3	5	9	14	23	37	57
45	0	1	1	2	3	4	7	12	20	33	48
40	0	0	0	1	1	3	5	10	19	32	46
35	0	0	0	1	1	2	4	8	15	29	44
30	0	0	0	0	1	2	3	6	12	24	43
25	0	0	0	0	1	1	3	6	11	22	42
20	0	0	0	0	0	1	1	3	7	15	33
15	0	0	0	0	0	0	0	1	2	4	8
10	0	0	0	0	0	0	0	0	1	2	3
5	0	0	0	0	0	0	0	0	0	0	0

Table 5.9. Fitted percentile scores for *Producción de Palabras* [Words Produced] (Inventario I)—boys

%ile rank	Age in months										
	8	9	10	11	12	13	14	15	16	17	18
99	20	30	43	61	85	116	154	195	238	280	316
95	12	18	26	38	55	77	106	141	181	224	266
90	7	9	13	18	25	35	48	65	86	112	143
85	5	7	9	13	18	25	35	47	64	85	111
80	3	5	6	9	13	18	25	34	47	63	84
75	3	4	5	7	10	14	18	25	34	45	60
70	2	3	4	5	8	11	15	20	28	37	51
65	2	2	3	5	6	9	12	16	22	29	49
60	2	2	3	4	5	7	9	13	17	29	46
55	0	1	1	1	2	4	7	11	18	28	46
50	0	0	1	1	2	3	6	9	16	27	44
45	0	0	1	1	2	3	5	8	14	24	39
40	0	0	0	0	1	1	3	5	9	17	32
35	0	0	0	0	0	1	2	4	8	15	30
30	0	0	0	0	0	1	1	3	7	15	26
25	0	0	0	0	0	0	1	2	5	10	22
20	0	0	0	0	0	0	1	2	4	8	17
15	0	0	0	0	0	0	1	1	2	5	11
10	0	0	0	0	0	0	0	0	0	1	1
5	0	0	0	0	0	0	0	0	0	0	0

Table 5.10. Fitted percentile scores for *Total de Gestos* [Total Gestures] (Inventario I)—both sexes combined

%ile rank	Age in months										
	8	**9**	**10**	**11**	**12**	**13**	**14**	**15**	**16**	**17**	**18**
99	37	43	47	51	55	57	59	61	62	63	64
95	31	35	39	43	47	50	53	55	57	59	60
90	25	29	33	38	42	46	49	52	55	57	59
85	24	27	31	36	39	43	46	49	52	54	56
80	22	25	29	33	37	40	44	47	50	53	55
75	20	23	27	31	34	38	42	45	48	51	53
70	18	21	24	28	32	36	40	44	47	50	52
65	16	19	23	26	30	34	38	41	45	48	51
60	15	18	21	24	28	32	36	40	43	47	50
55	14	16	20	23	27	30	34	38	42	45	48
50	13	15	18	22	25	29	33	37	40	44	47
45	12	14	17	20	24	28	31	35	39	43	46
40	11	14	16	19	23	26	30	34	37	41	44
35	11	13	15	18	21	25	28	32	36	39	43
30	9	11	14	16	19	23	27	30	34	38	42
25	8	10	12	15	18	21	24	28	32	36	39
20	7	9	11	13	16	19	22	26	30	34	38
15	6	8	9	12	14	17	21	24	28	32	36
10	5	6	7	9	11	14	17	21	25	29	33
5	2	3	4	5	7	10	13	17	22	27	32

Table 5.11. Fitted percentile scores for *Total de Gestos* [Total Gestures] (Inventario I)—girls

%ile rank	Age in months										
	8	9	10	11	12	13	14	15	16	17	18
99	35	41	46	51	54	57	59	61	62	63	64
95	32	37	42	46	50	53	56	58	60	61	62
90	27	32	36	40	44	48	51	54	56	58	59
85	24	28	33	37	41	45	49	52	54	57	58
80	22	26	30	34	39	43	47	50	53	55	57
75	20	24	28	32	36	40	44	47	50	53	55
70	18	22	26	30	34	38	42	46	49	52	54
65	17	20	23	27	31	35	39	43	47	50	52
60	15	19	22	26	30	34	38	42	45	48	51
55	14	17	21	25	28	32	37	40	44	47	51
50	13	16	19	22	26	30	34	38	42	46	49
45	12	15	18	21	25	29	33	37	41	44	48
40	12	15	18	21	24	28	32	36	39	43	46
35	11	14	16	19	23	27	30	34	38	42	45
30	10	12	15	18	21	24	28	32	36	40	43
25	9	11	13	16	19	22	26	30	33	37	41
20	8	10	12	15	17	21	24	28	31	35	39
15	6	8	10	12	15	18	22	26	30	34	38
10	5	6	8	10	12	15	19	22	27	31	35
5	0	2	5	8	11	13	16	19	22	24	27

Table 5.12. Fitted percentile scores for *Total de Gestos* [Total Gestures] (Inventario I)—boys

%ile rank	Age in months										
	8	9	10	11	12	13	14	15	16	17	18
99	34	38	42	46	49	52	54	57	58	60	61
95	28	33	37	41	44	48	51	54	56	58	59
90	26	30	33	37	40	43	46	49	52	54	56
85	22	26	29	33	37	40	44	47	49	52	54
80	21	24	28	31	35	39	42	45	48	51	53
75	20	23	27	30	34	37	41	44	47	50	52
70	18	21	24	27	31	35	38	42	45	48	50
65	15	18	21	25	29	33	37	40	44	47	50
60	14	17	20	23	27	31	35	38	42	45	48
55	13	16	18	22	25	29	33	37	40	44	47
50	13	15	18	21	25	28	32	35	39	42	46
45	12	15	17	20	23	26	30	33	37	40	43
40	11	13	16	19	22	25	29	32	36	39	43
35	10	12	14	17	20	24	27	31	35	38	42
30	8	10	12	15	18	21	25	29	33	37	41
25	7	9	11	13	16	20	23	27	31	35	39
20	7	8	10	12	15	18	21	25	29	33	37
15	6	7	9	11	13	16	19	23	27	31	35
10	4	5	7	9	11	14	17	20	24	28	33
5	3	4	5	6	8	10	12	15	19	23	27

Table 5.13. Fitted percentile scores for *Gestos Tempranos* [Early Gestures] (Inventario I)—both sexes combined

%ile rank	Age in months										
	8	9	10	11	12	13	14	15	16	17	18
99	19	19	20	20	20	20	21	21	21	21	21
95	17	17	18	19	19	20	20	21	21	21	21
90	13	15	16	17	18	19	20	20	21	21	21
85	13	14	15	16	17	18	18	19	20	20	20
80	12	13	15	15	16	17	18	19	19	20	20
75	12	13	14	15	16	16	17	18	18	19	19
70	11	12	13	14	15	16	17	18	18	19	19
65	11	12	13	14	15	16	16	17	18	18	19
60	10	11	12	13	14	15	16	17	17	18	19
55	10	11	12	13	14	15	16	16	17	18	18
50	10	11	12	12	13	14	15	16	17	17	18
45	9	10	11	12	13	14	15	15	16	17	17
40	8	9	10	11	12	13	14	15	16	16	17
35	8	9	10	11	12	13	13	14	15	16	17
30	7	8	9	10	11	12	13	14	14	15	16
25	7	8	9	9	10	11	12	13	14	15	16
20	6	7	8	9	10	11	11	12	13	14	15
15	5	6	7	8	9	9	10	11	12	13	14
10	4	5	6	7	8	9	10	11	12	13	14
5	2	3	4	4	5	6	8	9	10	12	13

Table 5.14. Fitted percentile scores for *Gestos Tempranos* [Early Gestures] (Inventario I)—girls

%ile rank	Age in months										
	8	9	10	11	12	13	14	15	16	17	18
99	19	19	19	20	20	20	21	21	21	21	21
95	18	19	19	19	20	20	20	21	21	21	21
90	15	16	17	18	19	19	20	20	21	21	21
85	13	14	16	17	18	19	19	20	20	21	21
80	13	14	15	16	17	18	18	19	19	20	20
75	12	13	14	15	16	17	18	18	19	19	20
70	12	13	14	15	15	16	17	18	18	19	19
65	11	12	13	14	15	16	17	18	18	19	19
60	11	12	13	14	15	16	16	17	18	19	19
55	11	12	12	13	14	15	16	16	17	18	18
50	10	11	12	13	14	15	15	16	17	17	18
45	9	10	11	12	13	14	15	16	16	17	18
40	9	10	11	12	13	14	14	15	16	17	17
35	8	9	10	11	12	13	14	15	15	16	17
30	8	8	9	10	11	12	13	14	15	16	17
25	7	8	9	10	11	12	13	14	15	16	16
20	7	7	8	9	10	11	12	13	14	15	15
15	6	7	7	8	9	10	11	12	13	14	15
10	5	5	6	7	8	9	10	11	12	13	14
5	2	3	4	5	6	7	8	9	10	11	12

Table 5.15. Fitted percentile scores for *Gestos Tempranos* [Early Gestures] (Inventario I)—boys

%ile rank	Age in months										
	8	9	10	11	12	13	14	15	16	17	18
99	17	18	19	19	20	20	20	21	21	21	21
95	15	16	17	18	19	19	20	20	21	21	21
90	14	15	16	17	18	18	19	19	20	20	21
85	13	14	15	16	17	17	18	19	19	20	20
80	12	13	14	15	16	17	18	18	19	19	20
75	12	13	14	15	15	16	17	18	18	19	19
70	11	12	13	14	15	16	16	17	18	18	19
65	11	12	13	14	15	15	16	17	18	18	19
60	10	11	12	13	14	15	16	17	17	18	19
55	9	10	11	12	13	14	15	16	17	17	18
50	9	10	11	12	13	14	15	16	16	17	18
45	9	10	10	11	12	13	14	15	16	16	17
40	8	9	10	11	12	12	13	14	15	16	16
35	7	8	9	10	11	12	13	14	14	15	16
30	7	8	9	9	10	11	12	13	14	15	15
25	7	7	8	9	10	11	11	12	13	14	15
20	5	6	7	8	9	10	11	12	13	14	15
15	5	6	7	7	8	9	10	11	12	13	14
10	4	4	5	6	7	8	9	10	11	12	14
5	2	3	4	4	5	6	7	8	10	11	12

Table 5.16. Fitted percentile scores for *Gestos Tardíos* [Later Gestures] (Inventario I)—both sexes combined

%ile rank	Age in months										
	8	**9**	**10**	**11**	**12**	**13**	**14**	**15**	**16**	**17**	**18**
99	21	25	29	32	35	37	39	41	42	42	43
95	16	19	22	25	28	31	34	36	37	39	40
90	13	15	18	21	25	28	31	33	35	37	39
85	12	14	17	20	23	26	29	31	34	36	37
80	9	12	14	17	20	24	27	30	32	35	37
75	9	11	13	16	19	22	25	28	30	33	35
70	7	9	12	15	18	20	23	26	29	32	34
65	5	7	10	13	16	19	21	24	27	30	32
60	4	7	9	12	15	18	21	23	26	29	32
55	3	6	9	11	14	17	20	22	25	28	31
50	3	5	8	11	13	16	19	21	24	26	29
45	1	4	7	9	12	15	17	20	23	25	28
40	0	3	6	8	11	13	16	19	21	24	27
35	0	3	5	8	10	13	15	18	20	23	25
30	0	2	5	7	9	11	14	16	18	21	23
25	0	2	4	6	8	11	13	15	17	20	22
20	0	1	3	5	7	10	12	14	16	18	20
15	0	0	2	4	6	8	10	12	14	16	18
10	0	0	1	3	5	7	9	10	12	14	16
5	0	0	1	2	4	5	6	8	9	11	12

Table 5.17. Fitted percentile scores for *Gestos Tardíos* [Later Gestures] (Inventario I)—girls

%ile rank	Age in months										
	8	**9**	**10**	**11**	**12**	**13**	**14**	**15**	**16**	**17**	**18**
99	19	23	27	31	34	37	39	40	42	42	43
95	18	21	25	28	31	34	36	38	40	41	42
90	14	17	20	23	26	29	32	34	36	38	39
85	12	14	17	21	24	27	30	33	35	37	39
80	11	13	16	19	22	25	28	30	33	36	39
75	8	11	14	17	20	23	26	29	32	34	37
70	7	10	13	16	18	21	24	27	30	33	36
65	6	9	12	15	17	20	23	26	29	32	35
60	5	7	10	13	16	19	22	25	28	31	34
55	4	7	10	13	15	18	21	24	27	29	32
50	3	6	9	11	14	17	20	22	25	28	31
45	2	5	8	11	13	16	19	22	25	27	30
40	1	4	7	9	12	15	17	20	23	26	28
35	1	3	6	9	11	14	17	19	22	24	27
30	0	3	5	8	10	13	15	18	20	23	25
25	0	2	5	7	9	12	14	16	19	21	23
20	0	1	4	6	8	10	12	14	17	19	21
15	0	0	2	4	6	8	10	12	14	17	19
10	0	0	2	3	5	7	9	11	13	15	17
5	0	0	0	2	4	5	7	9	10	12	14

Table 5.18. Fitted percentile scores for *Gestos Tardíos* [Later Gestures] (Inventario I)—boys

%ile rank	Age in months										
	8	**9**	**10**	**11**	**12**	**13**	**14**	**15**	**16**	**17**	**18**
99	17	21	25	29	33	35	38	39	41	42	42
95	15	18	21	24	27	30	33	35	37	38	39
90	13	15	18	21	23	26	29	32	34	36	37
85	10	13	15	18	21	24	27	30	32	34	36
80	9	12	15	17	20	22	25	28	30	33	35
75	8	11	13	16	18	21	24	26	29	31	34
70	6	9	11	14	17	19	22	25	27	30	33
65	5	7	10	12	15	18	20	23	26	28	31
60	4	6	9	11	14	17	19	22	25	27	30
55	3	5	8	11	13	16	18	21	23	26	29
50	2	5	7	10	12	15	17	20	22	25	27
45	1	4	6	9	11	14	16	19	21	24	26
40	1	3	5	8	10	13	15	18	20	23	25
35	0	2	5	7	9	12	14	16	19	21	23
30	0	2	4	6	9	11	13	16	18	20	23
25	0	2	4	6	8	10	12	14	16	18	21
20	0	1	3	5	7	9	11	13	15	17	19
15	0	0	2	4	6	8	10	12	13	15	17
10	0	0	2	3	5	6	8	9	11	13	14
5	0	0	1	2	4	5	6	7	9	10	11

Table 5.19. Fitted percentile scores for *Producción de Palabras* [Words Produced] (Inventario II)—both sexes combined

%ile rank	Age in months														
	16	**17**	**18**	**19**	**20**	**21**	**22**	**23**	**24**	**25**	**26**	**27**	**28**	**29**	**30**
99	566	592	613	630	642	652	659	665	669	672	674	676	677	678	679
95	261	308	357	404	449	491	527	558	584	606	623	636	647	655	661
90	181	217	257	299	343	387	429	468	504	535	563	586	605	621	634
85	151	181	215	252	291	332	373	413	451	486	518	546	570	590	608
80	131	157	185	217	251	287	324	362	400	435	469	500	528	553	575
75	110	132	158	187	218	253	290	327	366	403	439	473	504	532	556
70	89	108	131	157	186	219	254	291	330	369	407	444	478	509	537
65	71	88	108	131	159	189	224	261	300	340	381	420	457	491	522
60	59	73	90	111	135	163	195	230	268	307	348	389	428	465	499
55	52	64	79	97	119	144	173	205	240	278	318	358	398	436	472
50	43	54	67	83	102	124	150	180	214	250	289	330	371	411	449
45	35	45	56	69	86	106	130	157	188	223	260	300	341	382	422
40	29	36	46	58	72	90	112	137	166	200	236	276	318	360	402
35	26	33	42	52	65	80	98	120	146	175	208	244	282	322	363
30	22	28	36	45	56	70	86	106	129	156	187	222	259	299	339
25	19	24	30	37	47	58	72	89	109	132	159	190	224	261	300
20	16	20	25	31	39	49	61	75	93	114	138	167	198	234	271
15	12	15	19	23	29	36	45	55	68	84	102	123	148	176	207
10	10	12	15	18	22	27	34	41	50	61	74	90	108	129	152
5	6	7	9	11	14	17	21	25	31	38	46	56	68	82	99

Table 5.20. Fitted percentile scores for *Producción de Palabras* [Words Produced] (Inventario II)—girls

%ile rank	Age in months														
	16	17	18	19	20	21	22	23	24	25	26	27	28	29	30
99	499	540	574	601	622	638	650	658	665	669	673	675	677	678	679
95	272	329	388	443	494	537	572	600	622	638	650	659	665	670	673
90	194	237	283	332	382	429	473	513	547	576	599	618	633	644	653
85	161	198	239	284	330	377	423	466	504	538	567	591	610	626	639
80	129	158	192	230	271	315	359	403	445	483	518	548	573	595	613
75	116	140	168	200	235	272	311	351	391	429	465	498	528	554	576
70	109	130	154	182	212	244	279	315	352	388	423	457	488	516	542
65	86	104	125	150	177	208	242	277	315	352	390	426	461	493	521
60	71	86	105	127	153	182	214	249	286	325	364	402	439	474	505
55	60	74	90	110	133	160	190	224	260	298	338	377	416	452	486
50	48	60	74	92	112	136	164	195	229	267	306	346	386	425	462
45	43	54	66	81	99	120	144	172	203	237	273	311	350	388	426
40	38	47	58	71	87	106	128	154	183	215	251	288	327	366	404
35	28	35	45	56	70	88	109	133	162	195	232	271	313	355	397
30	23	29	37	47	60	75	94	117	143	174	209	248	289	332	375
25	20	26	33	41	53	66	83	103	128	156	189	225	265	307	350
20	16	20	26	33	41	52	64	80	99	121	148	178	212	249	288
15	13	17	21	26	33	41	52	64	79	98	119	144	173	206	241
10	11	14	17	21	26	32	39	48	58	71	85	103	123	146	172
5	6	7	9	12	15	18	23	29	36	45	56	69	85	104	126

Table 5.21. Fitted percentile scores for *Producción de Palabras* [Words Produced] (Inventario II)—boys

%ile rank	Age in months														
	16	17	18	19	20	21	22	23	24	25	26	27	28	29	30
99	446	479	509	535	559	579	597	612	624	635	643	651	656	661	665
95	287	323	360	397	432	465	496	524	549	570	589	605	619	630	639
90	196	229	264	301	339	377	414	449	482	512	539	562	582	600	614
85	132	159	190	224	261	300	340	380	419	456	491	521	548	572	592
80	105	128	155	186	220	257	297	337	378	418	455	490	521	549	572
75	88	108	132	159	190	224	262	301	342	382	422	459	493	524	551
70	70	88	108	132	161	193	228	267	308	349	391	431	468	503	533
65	56	70	88	109	135	165	198	236	277	320	363	406	446	484	518
60	48	61	76	95	118	144	175	209	248	288	331	374	415	455	491
55	44	56	70	87	107	131	159	191	226	265	306	347	389	429	466
50	34	43	55	69	86	106	131	160	192	229	269	311	353	396	436
45	31	39	49	61	76	93	114	138	166	197	232	269	309	349	389
40	28	36	44	55	68	84	103	126	152	181	214	250	288	328	368
35	25	32	39	49	60	74	91	110	133	159	189	222	258	295	334
30	22	28	34	43	53	65	79	96	117	140	167	197	230	266	303
25	19	24	29	36	45	55	67	82	100	120	144	171	201	234	269
20	15	19	23	29	36	45	55	68	83	102	123	148	176	208	242
15	11	14	17	21	26	32	40	49	61	74	90	109	131	157	185
10	8	10	12	15	19	23	28	34	41	50	60	72	86	103	122
5	5	6	7	9	10	13	15	19	23	28	34	41	49	60	71

Table 5.22. Fitted percentile scores for *M3L-Palabras* [M3L-*Words] (Inventario II)—both sexes combined

%ile rank	Age in months														
	16	**17**	**18**	**19**	**20**	**21**	**22**	**23**	**24**	**25**	**26**	**27**	**28**	**29**	**30**
99	4	5	5	6	7	8	9	10	10	11	11	12	12	12	12
95	2	3	3	4	4	5	5	6	7	7	8	8	9	10	10
90	2	2	3	3	3	4	4	5	5	6	7	7	8	8	9
85	2	2	2	3	3	3	4	4	5	5	6	6	7	7	8
80	2	2	2	3	3	3	4	4	4	5	5	6	6	6	7
75	2	2	2	2	3	3	3	4	4	4	5	5	5	6	6
70	2	2	2	2	2	3	3	3	4	4	4	5	5	5	6
65	1	2	2	2	2	2	3	3	3	4	4	5	5	5	6
60	1	1	1	2	2	2	2	3	3	3	4	4	5	5	6
55	1	1	1	2	2	2	2	3	3	3	4	4	5	5	5
50	1	1	1	1	2	2	2	2	3	3	3	4	4	5	5
45	1	1	1	1	1	2	2	2	2	3	3	3	4	4	5
40	1	1	1	1	1	2	2	2	2	3	3	3	4	4	4
35	1	1	1	1	1	1	2	2	2	2	3	3	3	4	4
30	1	1	1	1	1	1	2	2	2	2	2	3	3	3	4
25	1	1	1	1	1	1	1	2	2	2	2	2	3	3	3
20	1	1	1	1	1	1	1	1	2	2	2	2	2	2	3
15	1	1	1	1	1	1	1	1	1	2	2	2	2	2	2
10	1	1	1	1	1	1	1	1	1	1	1	1	2	2	2
5	1	1	1	1	1	1	1	1	1	1	1	1	1	1	1

Table 5.23. Fitted percentile scores for *M3L-Palabras* [M3L-*Words] (Inventario II)—girls

%ile rank	Age in months														
	16	17	18	19	20	21	22	23	24	25	26	27	28	29	30
99	4	5	5	6	7	8	9	9	10	11	11	12	12	12	12
95	3	3	4	5	5	6	7	8	8	9	10	10	11	11	12
90	2	2	3	3	4	4	5	5	6	6	7	8	8	9	9
85	2	2	3	3	3	4	4	5	5	6	6	7	7	8	8
80	2	2	2	3	3	3	4	4	5	5	6	6	7	7	8
75	2	2	2	3	3	3	4	4	4	5	5	6	6	7	7
70	2	2	2	2	3	3	3	4	4	5	5	5	6	6	7
65	2	2	2	2	2	3	3	3	4	4	4	5	5	6	6
60	1	2	2	2	2	3	3	3	3	4	4	5	5	5	6
55	1	1	1	2	2	2	2	3	3	4	4	4	5	5	6
50	1	1	1	1	2	2	2	3	3	3	4	4	5	5	6
45	1	1	1	1	2	2	2	2	3	3	3	4	4	5	5
40	1	1	1	1	2	2	2	2	3	3	3	4	4	4	5
35	1	1	1	1	1	2	2	2	2	3	3	3	4	4	5
30	1	1	1	1	1	1	2	2	2	2	3	3	3	4	4
25	1	1	1	1	1	1	2	2	2	2	2	3	3	3	4
20	1	1	1	1	1	1	1	2	2	2	2	2	3	3	3
15	1	1	1	1	1	1	1	1	1	2	2	2	2	2	2
10	1	1	1	1	1	1	1	1	1	1	2	2	2	2	2
5	1	1	1	1	1	1	1	1	1	1	1	1	1	1	1

Table 5.24. Fitted percentile scores for *M3L-Palabras* [M3L-*Words] (Inventario II)—boys

%ile rank	Age in months														
	16	17	18	19	20	21	22	23	24	25	26	27	28	29	30
99	3	3	4	5	5	6	7	7	8	9	9	10	10	11	11
95	3	3	3	4	4	5	5	6	6	7	8	8	9	9	10
90	2	2	3	3	3	4	4	4	5	5	6	6	7	7	8
85	2	2	2	3	3	3	3	4	4	4	5	5	6	6	6
80	2	2	2	2	3	3	3	4	4	4	5	5	5	6	6
75	2	2	2	2	2	3	3	3	4	4	4	5	5	5	6
70	1	2	2	2	2	2	3	3	3	4	4	4	5	5	6
65	1	1	2	2	2	2	3	3	3	4	4	4	5	5	6
60	1	1	1	1	2	2	2	2	3	3	4	4	4	5	5
55	1	1	1	1	2	2	2	2	3	3	3	4	4	5	5
50	1	1	1	1	1	2	2	2	2	3	3	3	4	4	5
45	1	1	1	1	1	2	2	2	2	3	3	3	4	4	4
40	1	1	1	1	1	2	2	2	2	2	3	3	3	4	4
35	1	1	1	1	1	2	2	2	2	2	3	3	3	3	4
30	1	1	1	1	1	1	2	2	2	2	2	3	3	3	3
25	1	1	1	1	1	1	1	1	2	2	2	2	2	2	3
20	1	1	1	1	1	1	1	1	2	2	2	2	2	2	2
15	1	1	1	1	1	1	1	1	1	1	2	2	2	2	2
10	1	1	1	1	1	1	1	1	1	1	1	1	1	1	1
5	1	1	1	1	1	1	1	1	1	1	1	1	1	1	1

Table 5.25. Fitted percentile scores for *Complejidad de Frases* [Complexity] (Inventario II)—both sexes combined

%ile rank	Age in months														
	16	**17**	**18**	**19**	**20**	**21**	**22**	**23**	**24**	**25**	**26**	**27**	**28**	**29**	**30**
99	27	29	30	32	33	34	35	35	36	36	37	37	37	37	37
95	3	4	7	9	13	17	21	26	29	32	34	35	36	37	37
90	1	1	2	3	4	7	11	16	21	26	30	33	35	37	37
85	0	0	0	0	0	1	3	5	11	18	26	32	35	37	37
80	0	0	0	0	0	1	2	4	7	13	20	27	32	35	37
75	0	0	0	0	0	1	1	3	5	9	15	22	28	32	35
70	0	0	0	0	0	0	1	1	3	6	11	17	25	31	34
65	0	0	0	0	0	0	0	1	2	4	8	14	21	28	32
60	0	0	0	0	0	0	0	1	2	3	6	10	17	23	29
55	0	0	0	0	0	0	0	0	1	2	4	7	12	18	25
50	0	0	0	0	0	0	0	0	0	1	2	3	6	10	16
45	0	0	0	0	0	0	0	0	0	1	1	3	5	8	14
40	0	0	0	0	0	0	0	0	0	0	1	1	2	4	7
35	0	0	0	0	0	0	0	0	0	0	0	1	1	2	3
30	0	0	0	0	0	0	0	0	0	0	0	0	1	1	1
25	0	0	0	0	0	0	0	0	0	0	0	0	0	1	1
20	0	0	0	0	0	0	0	0	0	0	0	0	0	0	0
15	0	0	0	0	0	0	0	0	0	0	0	0	0	0	0
10	0	0	0	0	0	0	0	0	0	0	0	0	0	0	0
5	0	0	0	0	0	0	0	0	0	0	0	0	0	0	0

Table 5.26. Fitted percentile scores for *Complejidad de Frases* [Complexity] (Inventario II)—girls

%ile rank	Age in months														
	16	17	18	19	20	21	22	23	24	25	26	27	28	29	30
99	24	27	29	30	32	33	34	35	35	36	36	37	37	37	37
95	4	6	9	12	16	20	24	28	31	33	35	36	37	37	37
90	1	1	2	3	5	9	13	19	24	29	32	35	36	37	37
85	0	0	0	1	2	3	6	10	16	23	29	33	35	37	37
80	0	0	0	0	0	1	2	5	10	18	26	31	35	37	37
75	0	0	0	0	0	1	2	4	7	13	20	27	32	35	36
70	0	0	0	0	0	1	1	2	5	9	15	22	28	33	35
65	0	0	0	0	0	0	1	1	3	5	10	17	24	30	34
60	0	0	0	0	0	0	0	1	2	4	8	14	21	28	33
55	0	0	0	0	0	0	0	1	1	2	5	9	16	23	29
50	0	0	0	0	0	0	0	0	1	1	2	4	8	14	20
45	0	0	0	0	0	0	0	0	0	1	2	4	7	11	18
40	0	0	0	0	0	0	0	0	0	1	1	3	5	9	14
35	0	0	0	0	0	0	0	0	0	0	1	1	2	3	5
30	0	0	0	0	0	0	0	0	0	0	0	0	1	1	2
25	0	0	0	0	0	0	0	0	0	0	0	0	1	1	2
20	0	0	0	0	0	0	0	0	0	0	0	0	0	0	0
15	0	0	0	0	0	0	0	0	0	0	0	0	0	0	0
10	0	0	0	0	0	0	0	0	0	0	0	0	0	0	0
5	0	0	0	0	0	0	0	0	0	0	0	0	0	0	0

Table 5.27. Fitted percentile scores for *Complejidad de Frases* [Complexity] (Inventario II)—boys

%ile rank	Age in months														
	16	17	18	19	20	21	22	23	24	25	26	27	28	29	30
99	12	15	18	21	25	27	30	32	33	35	36	36	37	37	37
95	3	5	7	10	13	17	21	25	28	31	33	35	36	37	37
90	0	0	1	1	2	4	6	11	17	23	29	33	35	36	37
85	0	0	0	0	1	2	3	6	10	16	23	29	33	35	36
80	0	0	0	0	0	1	2	3	6	10	16	23	29	33	35
75	0	0	0	0	0	0	1	2	3	6	11	18	25	30	34
70	0	0	0	0	0	0	1	1	2	4	8	14	21	27	32
65	0	0	0	0	0	0	0	1	2	3	6	10	17	23	29
60	0	0	0	0	0	0	0	1	1	2	5	8	13	20	26
55	0	0	0	0	0	0	0	1	1	2	4	6	11	16	22
50	0	0	0	0	0	0	0	0	0	1	2	3	5	9	15
45	0	0	0	0	0	0	0	0	0	1	1	2	3	6	10
40	0	0	0	0	0	0	0	0	0	0	0	1	1	2	4
35	0	0	0	0	0	0	0	0	0	0	0	1	1	1	2
30	0	0	0	0	0	0	0	0	0	0	0	0	0	1	1
25	0	0	0	0	0	0	0	0	0	0	0	0	0	0	0
20	0	0	0	0	0	0	0	0	0	0	0	0	0	0	0
15	0	0	0	0	0	0	0	0	0	0	0	0	0	0	0
10	0	0	0	0	0	0	0	0	0	0	0	0	0	0	0
5	0	0	0	0	0	0	0	0	0	0	0	0	0	0	0

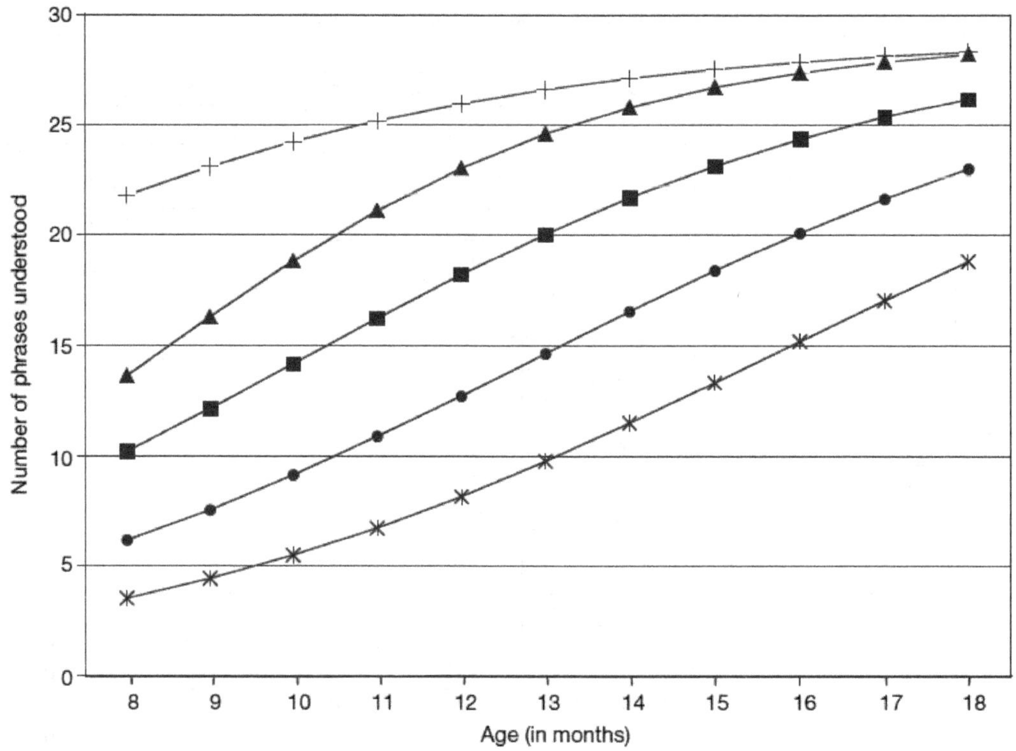

Figure 5.1. *Comprensión de las Primeras Frases* [Phrases Understood] (Inventario I)—both sexes combined. (*Key:* —+— 90th percentile; —▲— 75th percentile; —■— 50th percentile; —●—25th percentile; —✳— 10th percentile.)

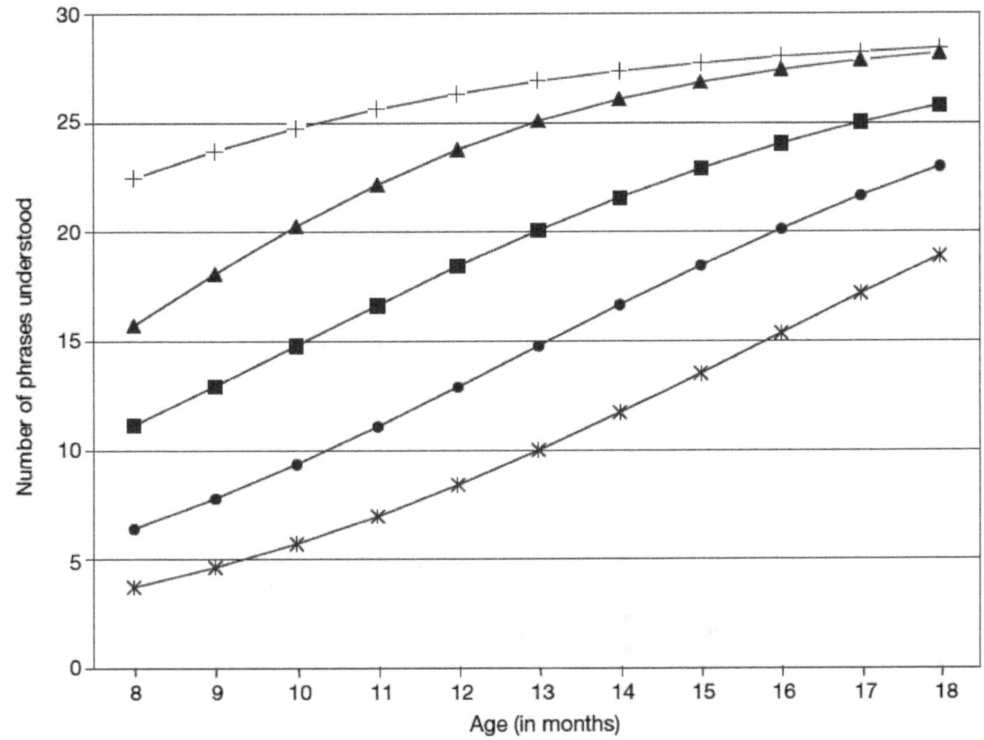

Figure 5.2. *Comprensión de las Primeras Frases* [Phrases Understood] (Inventario I)—girls. (*Key:* —+— 90th percentile; —▲— 75th percentile; —■— 50th percentile; —●—25th percentile; —✳— 10th percentile.)

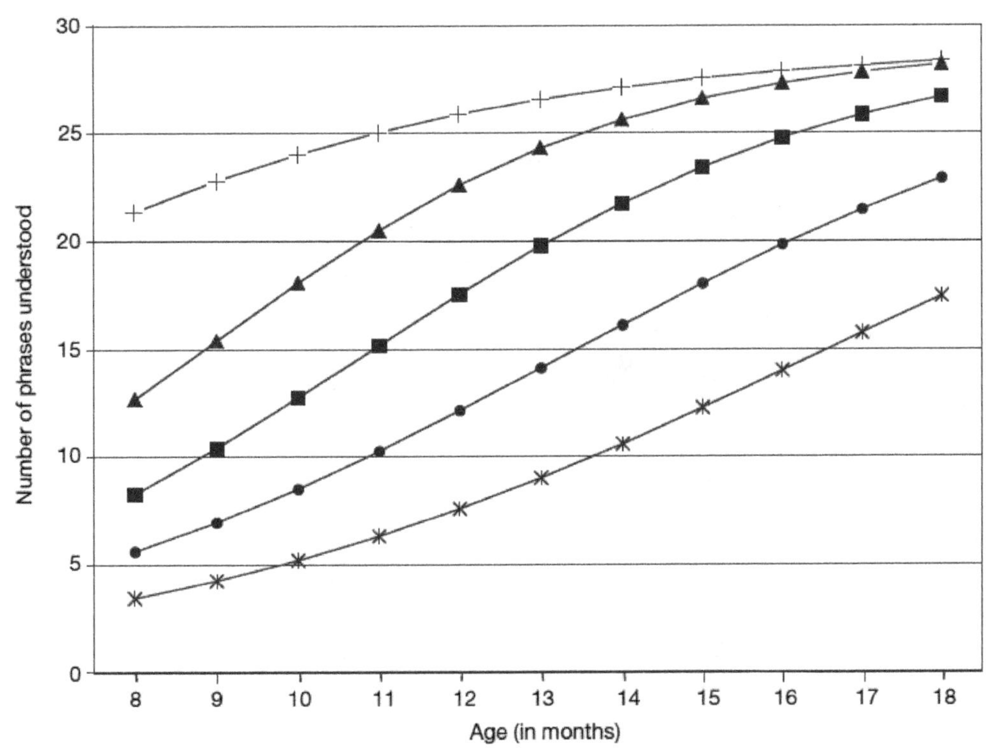

Figure 5.3. *Comprensión de las Primeras Frases* [Phrases Understood] (Inventario I)—boys. (*Key:* —+— 90th percentile; —▲— 75th percentile; —■— 50th percentile; —●—25th percentile; —✳— 10th percentile.)

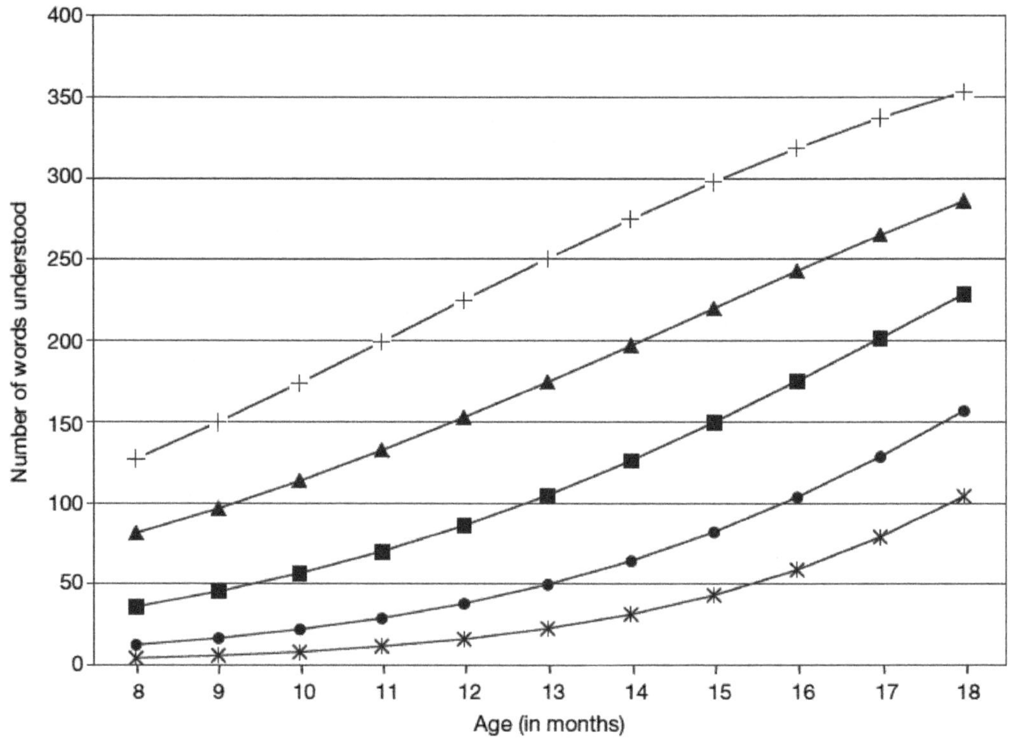

Figure 5.4. *Comprensión de Palabras* [Words Understood] (Inventario I)—both sexes combined. (*Key:* —+— 90th percentile; —▲— 75th percentile; —■— 50th percentile; —●—25th percentile; —✱— 10th percentile.)

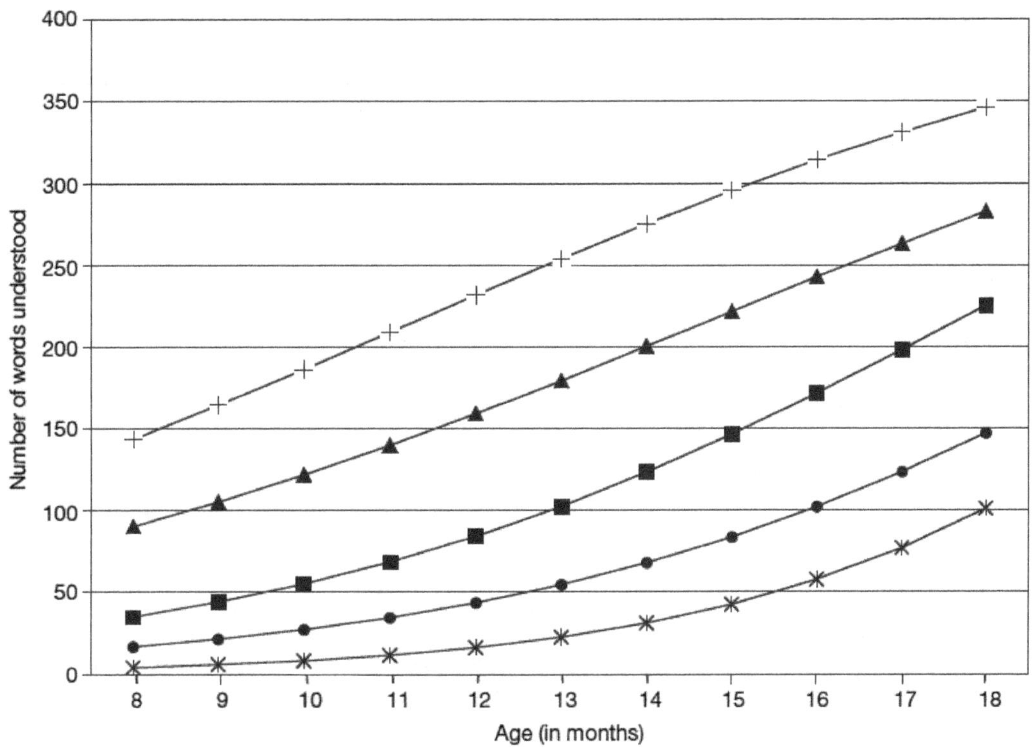

Figure 5.5. *Comprensión de Palabras* [Words Understood] (Inventario I)—girls. (*Key:* —+— 90th percentile; —▲— 75th percentile; —■— 50th percentile; —●—25th percentile; —✱— 10th percentile.)

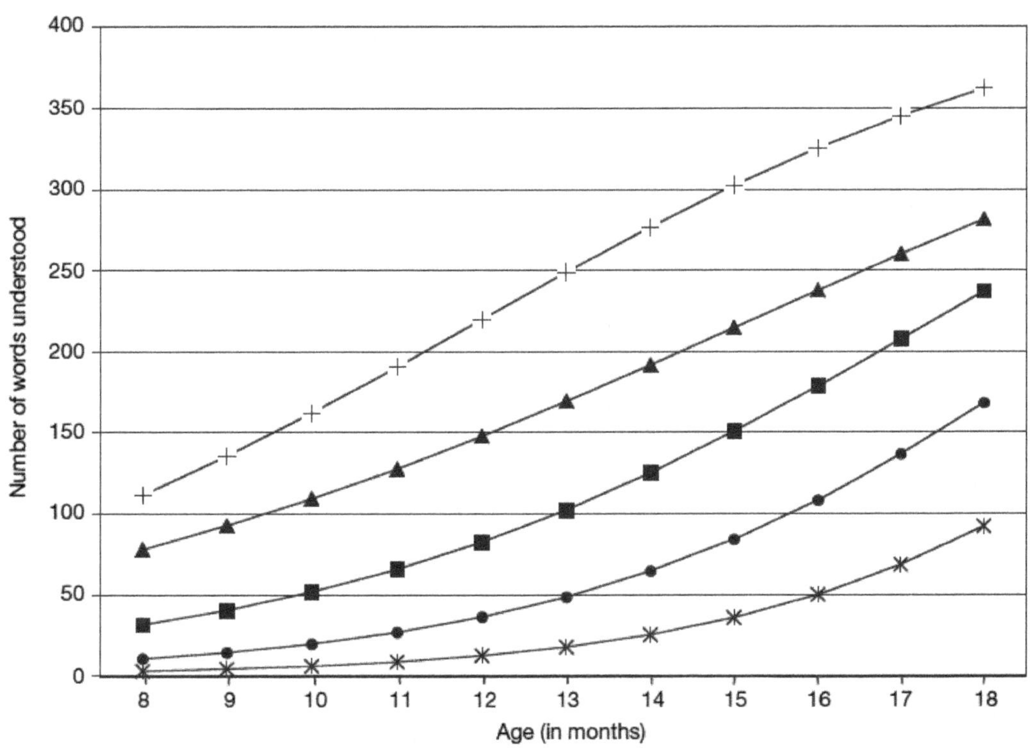

Figure 5.6. *Comprensión de Palabras* [Words Understood] (Inventario I)—boys. (*Key:* —+— 90th percentile; —▲— 75th percentile; —■— 50th percentile; —●—25th percentile; —✱— 10th percentile.)

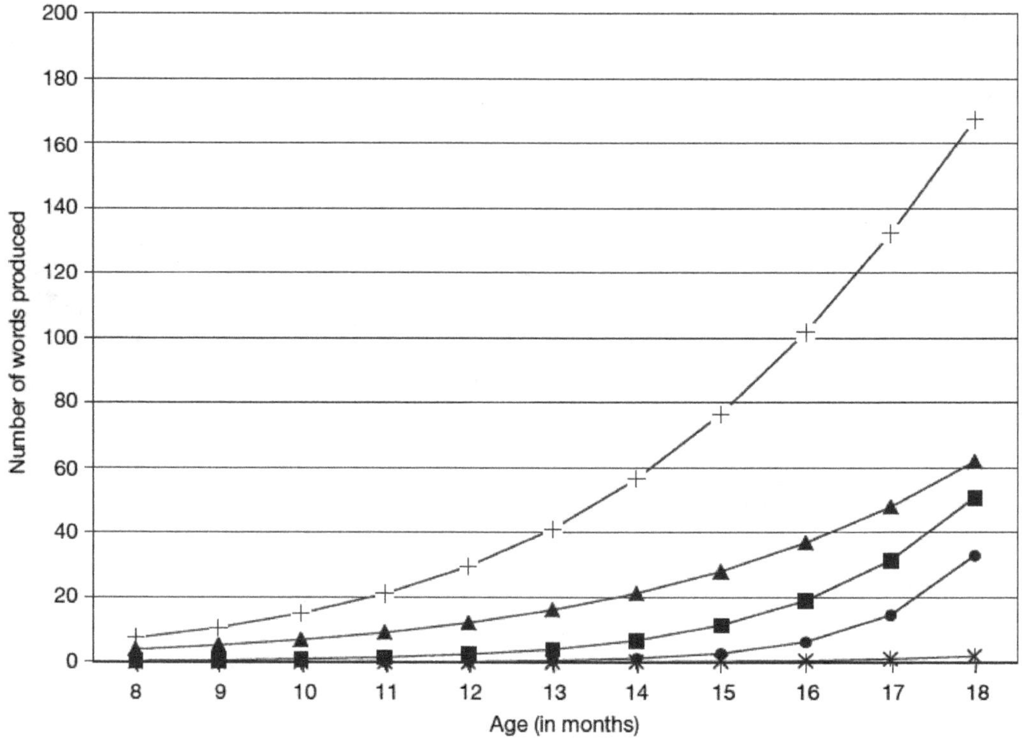

Figure 5.7. *Producción de Palabras* [Words Produced] (Inventario I)—both sexes combined. (*Key:* —+— 90th percentile; —▲— 75th percentile; —■— 50th percentile; —●—25th percentile; —✱— 10th percentile.)

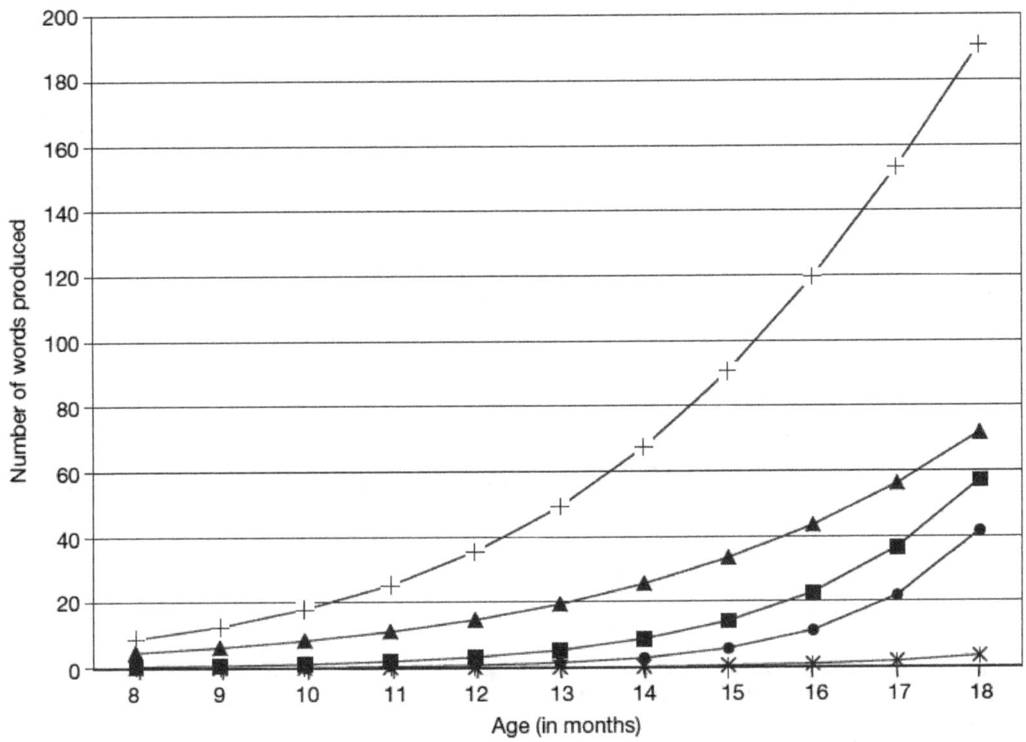

Figure 5.8. *Producción de Palabras* [Words Produced] (Inventario I)—girls. (*Key:* —+— 90th percentile; —▲— 75th percentile; —■— 50th percentile; —●—25th percentile; —✳— 10th percentile.)

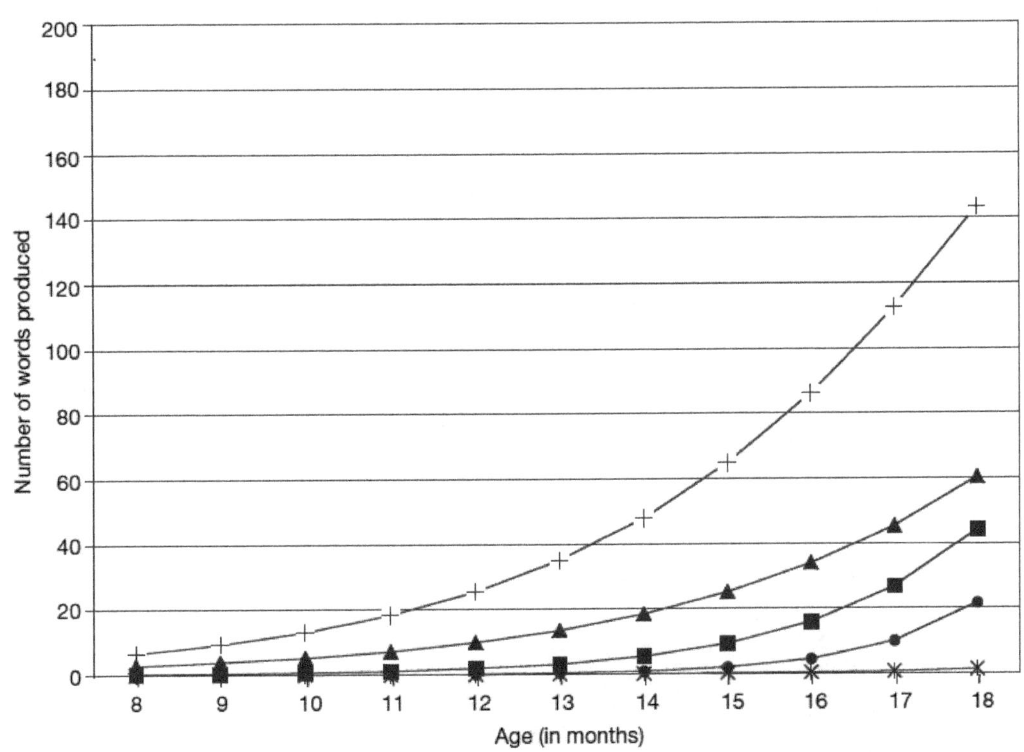

Figure 5.9. *Producción de Palabras* [Words Produced] (Inventario I)—boys. (*Key:* —+— 90th percentile; —▲— 75th percentile; —■— 50th percentile; —●—25th percentile; —✳— 10th percentile.)

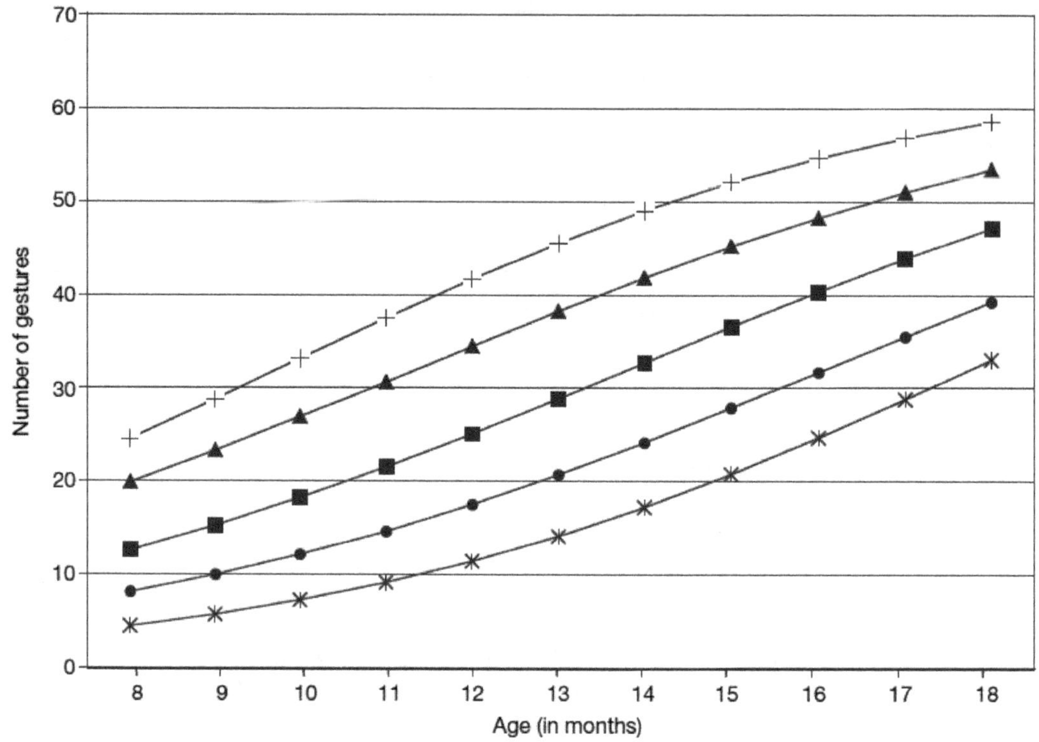

Figure 5.10. *Total de Gestos* [Total Gestures] (Inventario I)—both sexes combined. (*Key:* —+— 90th percentile; —▲— 75th percentile; —■— 50th percentile; —●—25th percentile; —✳— 10th percentile.)

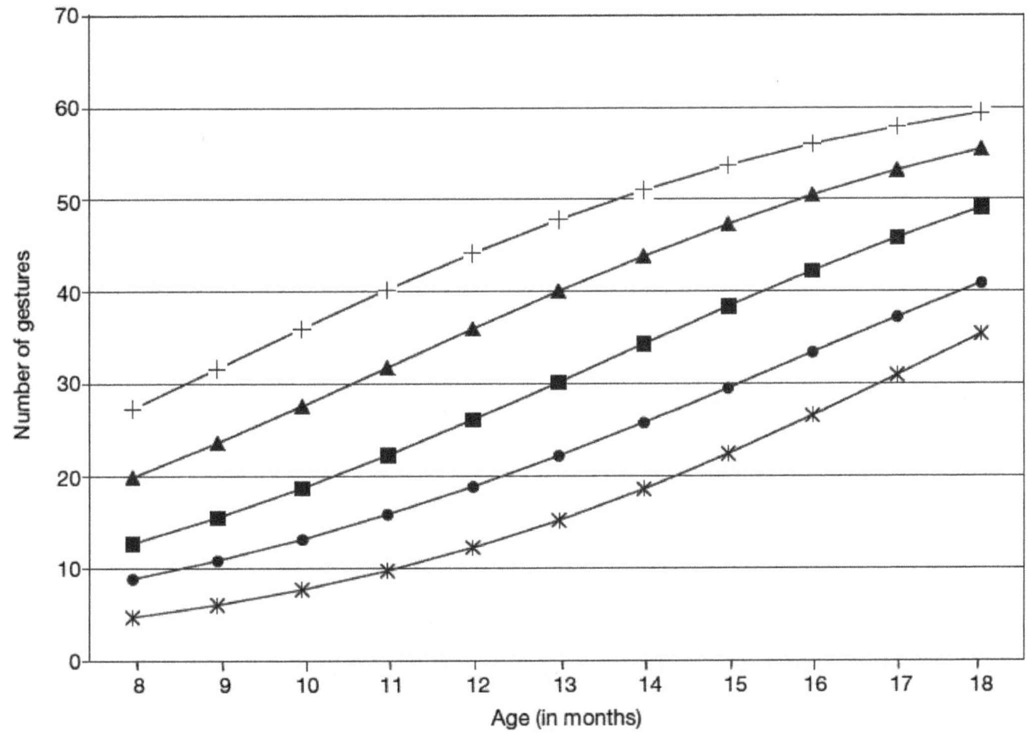

Figure 5.11. *Total de Gestos* [Total Gestures] (Inventario I)—girls. (*Key:* —+— 90th percentile; —▲— 75th percentile; —■— 50th percentile; —●—25th percentile; —✱— 10th percentile.)

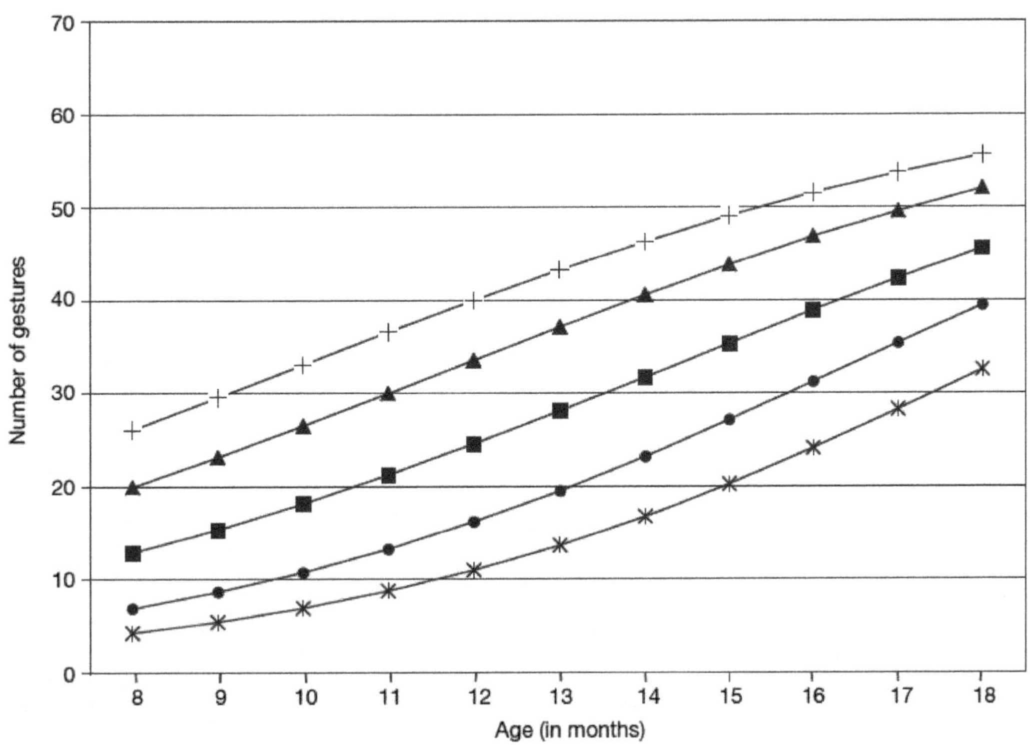

Figure 5.12. *Total de Gestos* [Total Gestures] (Inventario I)—boys. (*Key:* —+— 90th percentile; —▲— 75th percentile; —■— 50th percentile; —●—25th percentile; —✱— 10th percentile.)

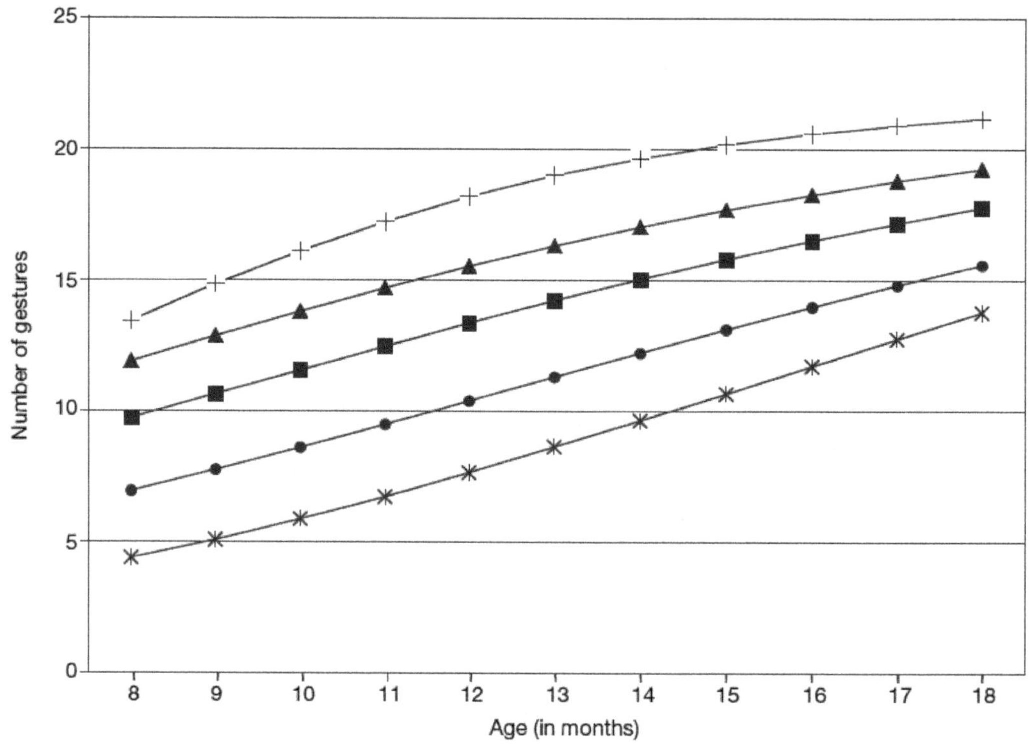

Figure 5.13. *Gestos Tempranos* [Early Gestures] (Inventario I)—both sexes combined. (*Key:* —+— 90th percentile; —▲— 75th percentile; —■— 50th percentile; —●—25th percentile; —✱— 10th percentile.)

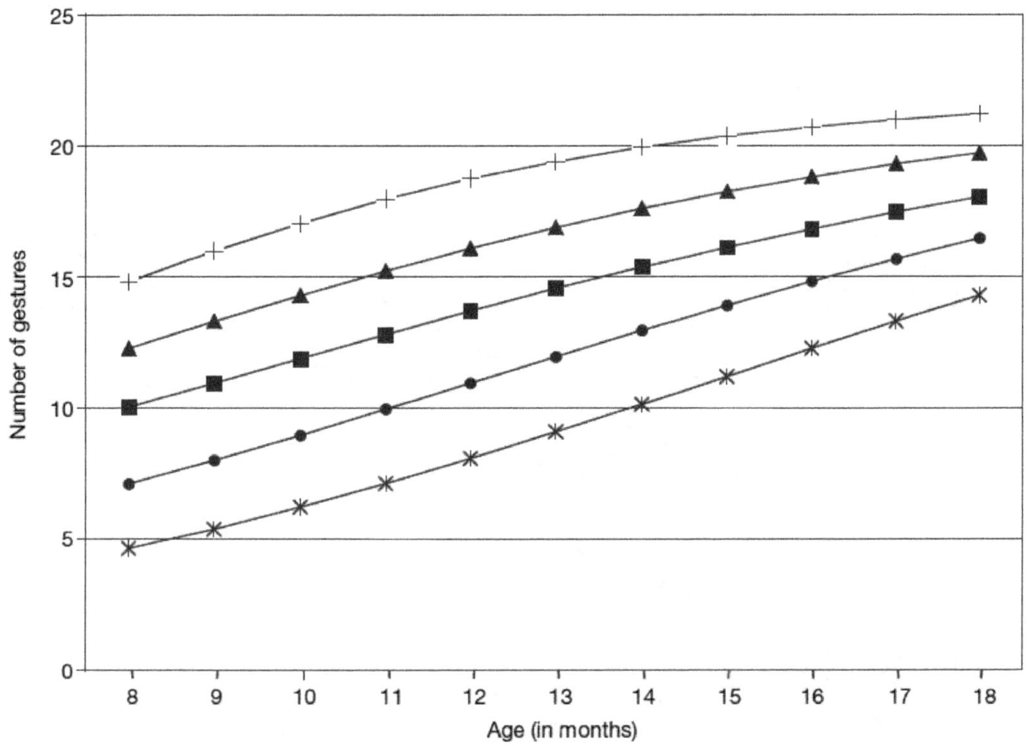

Figure 5.14. *Gestos Tempranos* [Early Gestures] (Inventario I)—girls. (*Key:* —+— 90th percentile; —▲— 75th percentile; —■— 50th percentile; —●—25th percentile; —✳— 10th percentile.)

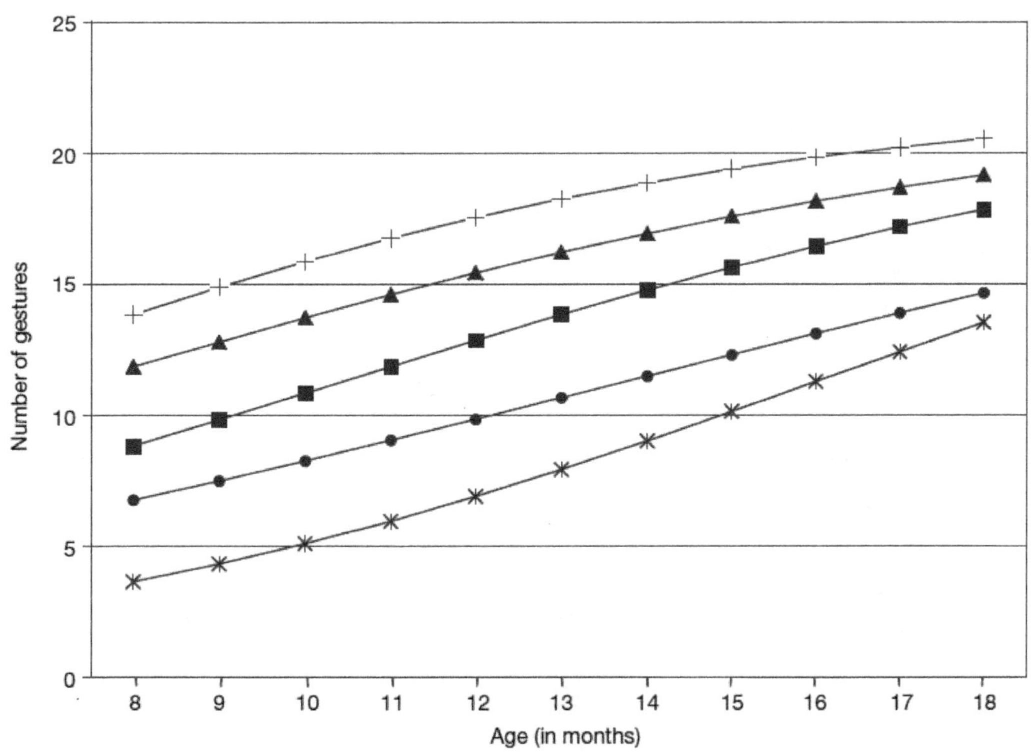

Figure 5.15. *Gestos Tempranos* [Early Gestures] (Inventario I)—boys. (*Key:* —+— 90th percentile; —▲— 75th percentile; —■— 50th percentile; —●—25th percentile; —✳— 10th percentile.)

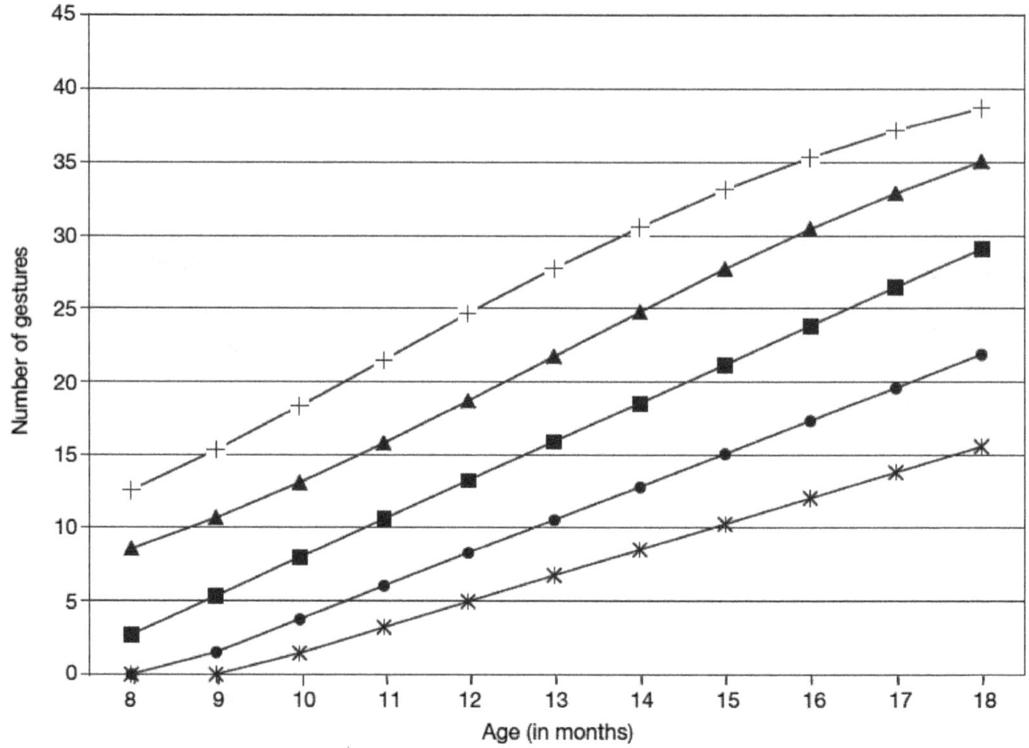

Figure 5.16. *Gestos Tardíos* [Later Gestures] (Inventario I)—both sexes combined. (*Key:* —+— 90th percentile; —▲— 75th percentile; —■— 50th percentile; —●—25th percentile; —✱— 10th percentile.)

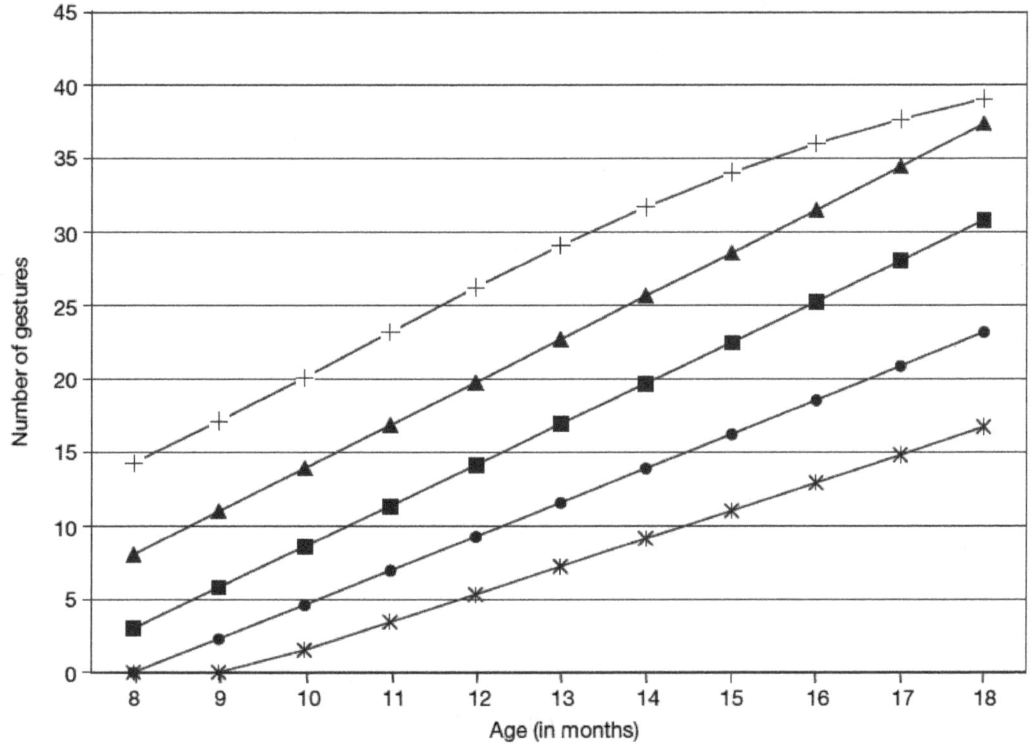

Figure 5.17. *Gestos Tardíos* [Later Gestures] (Inventario I)—girls. (*Key:* —+— 90th percentile; —▲— 75th percentile; —■— 50th percentile; —●—25th percentile; —✳— 10th percentile.)

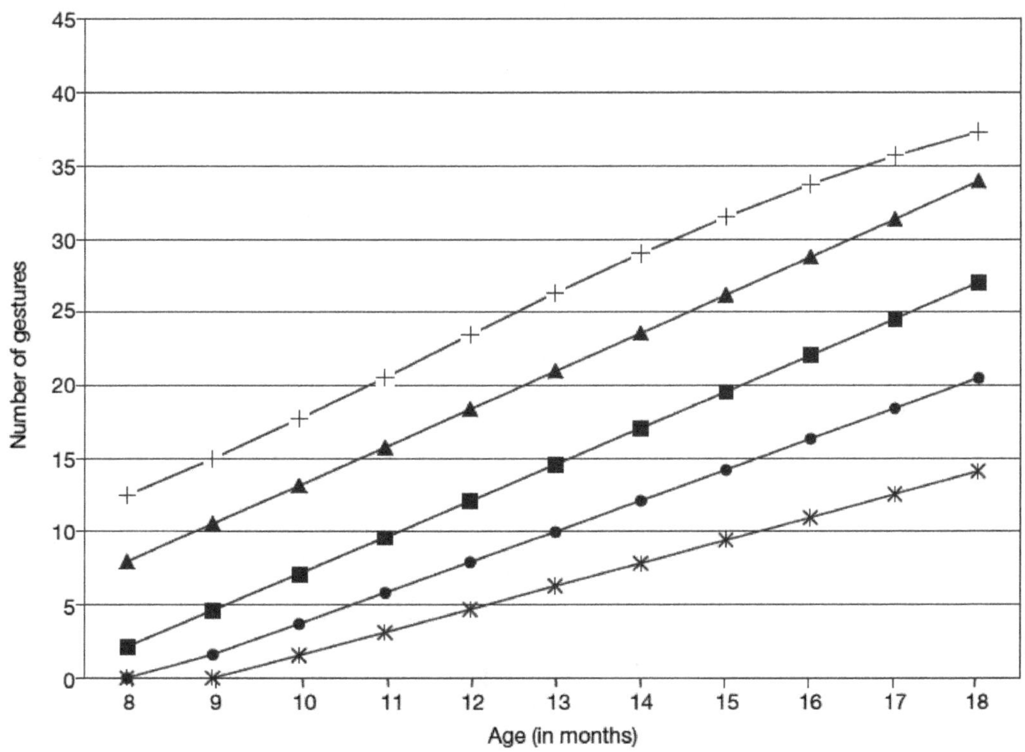

Figure 5.18. *Gestos Tardíos* [Later Gestures] (Inventario I)—boys. (*Key:* —+— 90th percentile; —▲— 75th percentile; —■— 50th percentile; —●—25th percentile; —✳— 10th percentile.)

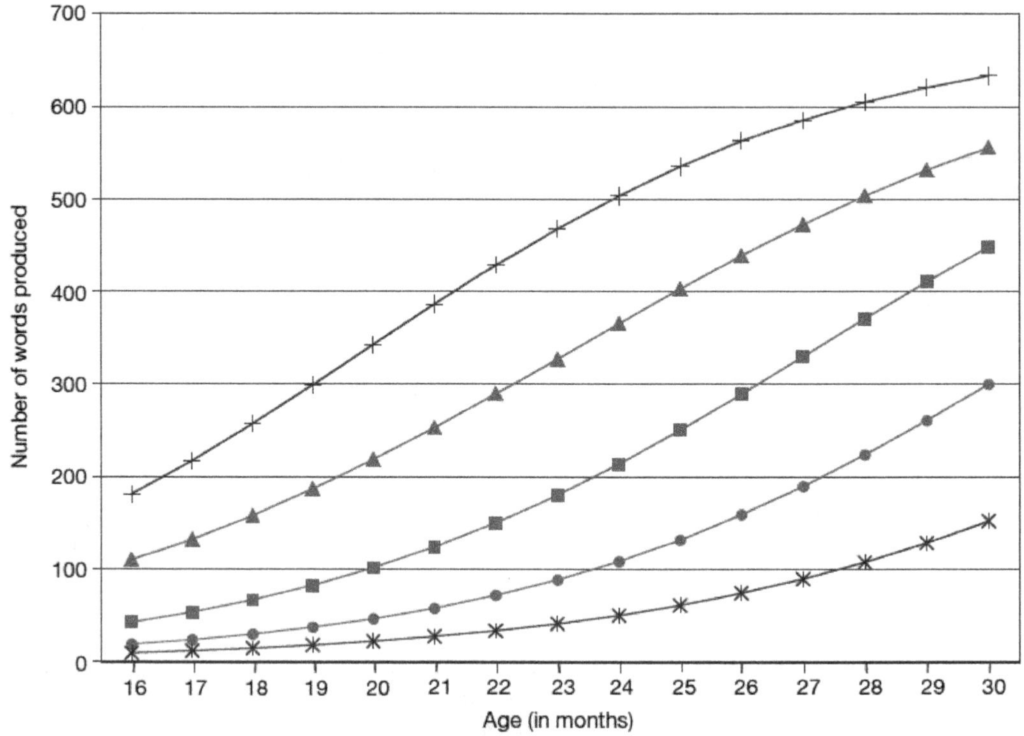

Figure 5.19. *Producción de Palabras* [Words Produced] (Inventario II)—both sexes combined. (*Key:* —+— 90th percentile; —▲— 75th percentile; —■— 50th percentile; —●—25th percentile; —✳— 10th percentile.)

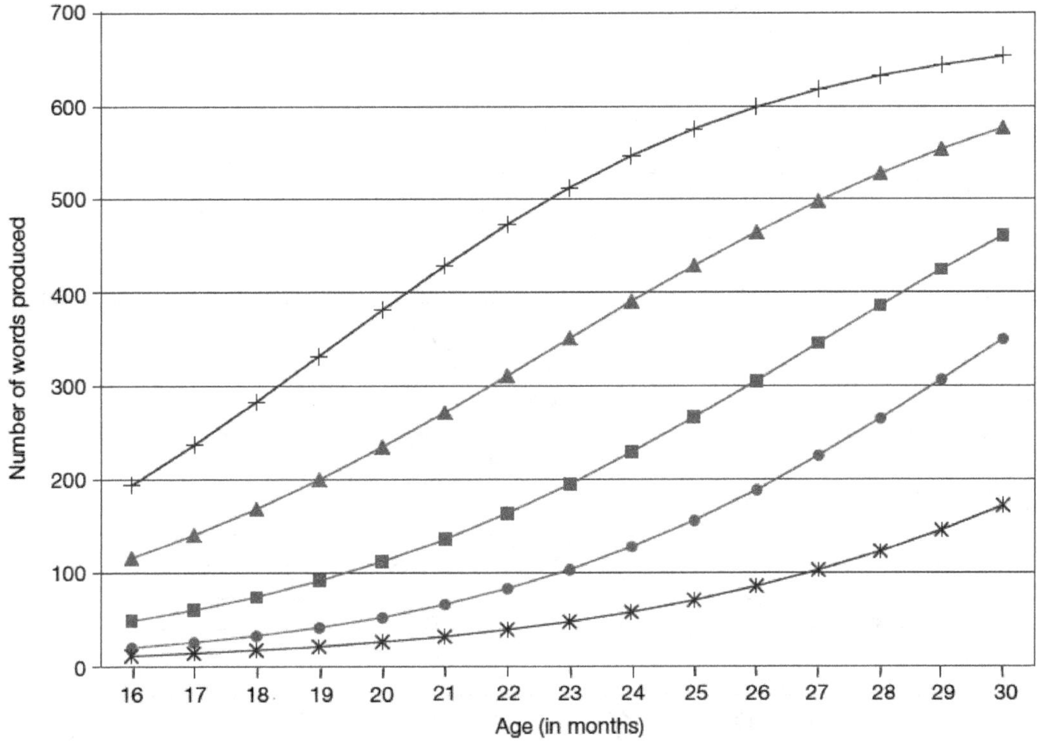

Figure 5.20. *Producción de Palabras* [Words Produced] (Inventario II)—girls. (*Key:* —+— 90th percentile; —▲— 75th percentile; —■— 50th percentile; —●—25th percentile; —✳— 10th percentile.)

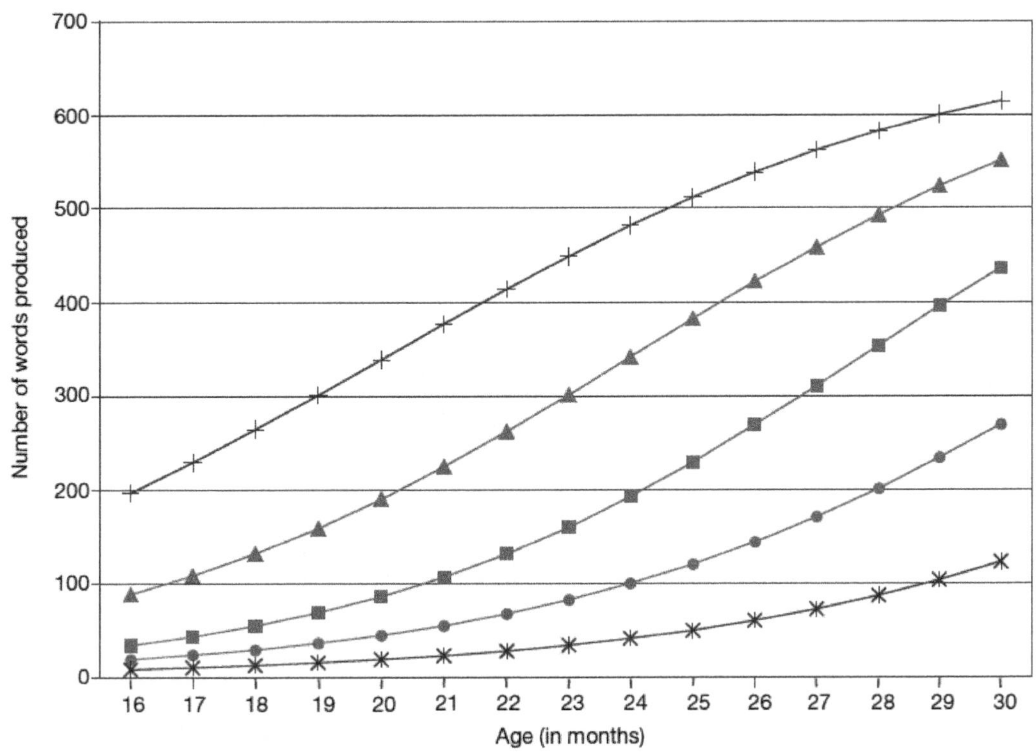

Figure 5.21. *Producción de Palabras* [Words Produced] (Inventario II)—boys. (*Key:* —+— 90th percentile; —▲— 75th percentile; —■— 50th percentile; —●—25th percentile; —✳— 10th percentile.)

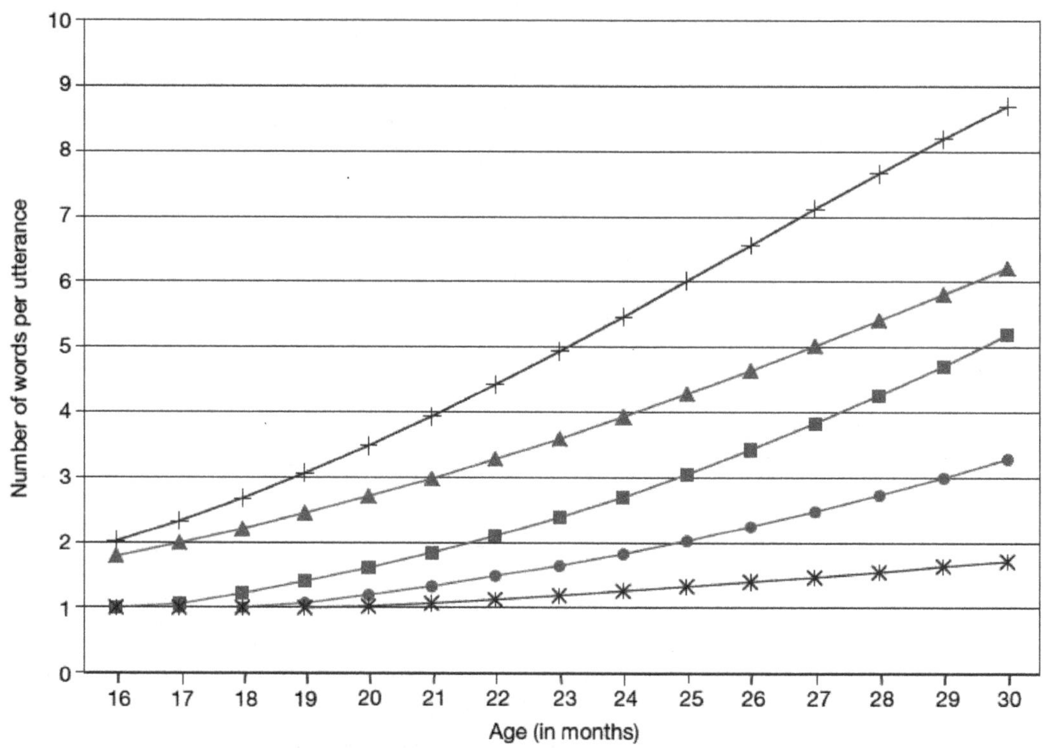

Figure 5.22. *M3L-Palabras* [M3L-"Words] (Inventario II)—both sexes combined. (*Key:* —+— 90th percentile; —▲— 75th percentile; —■— 50th percentile; —●—25th percentile; —✳— 10th percentile.)

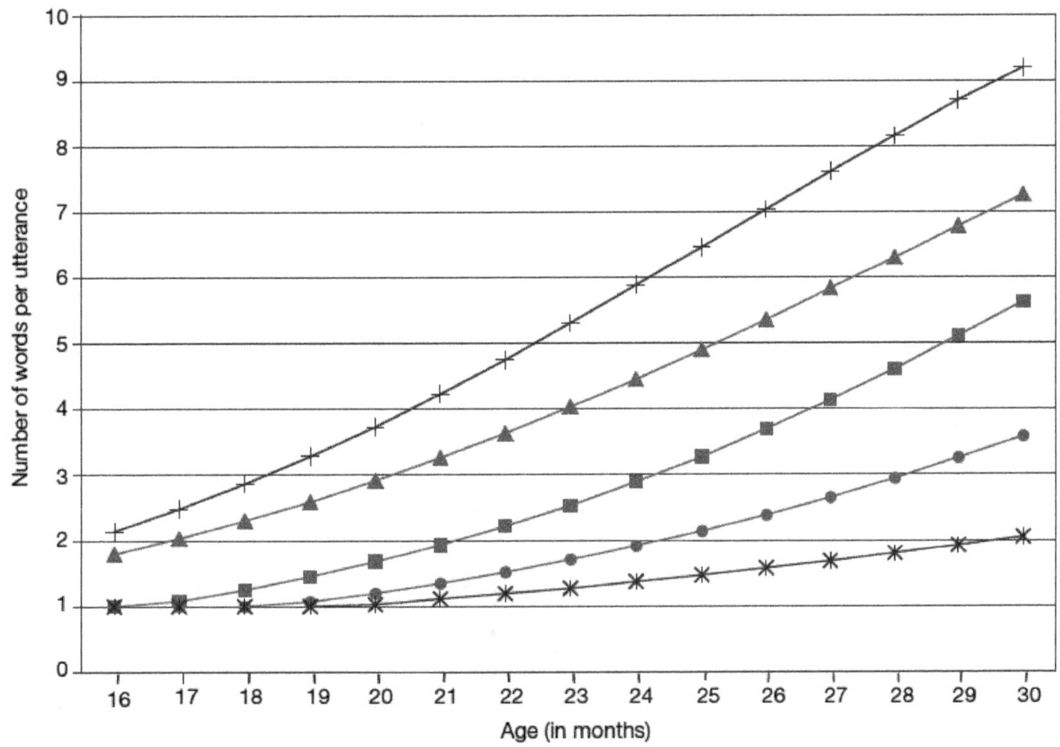

Figure 5.23. *M3L-Palabras* [M3L-*Words] (Inventario II)—girls. (*Key:* —+— 90th percentile; —▲— 75th percentile; —■— 50th percentile; —●—25th percentile; —✳— 10th percentile.)

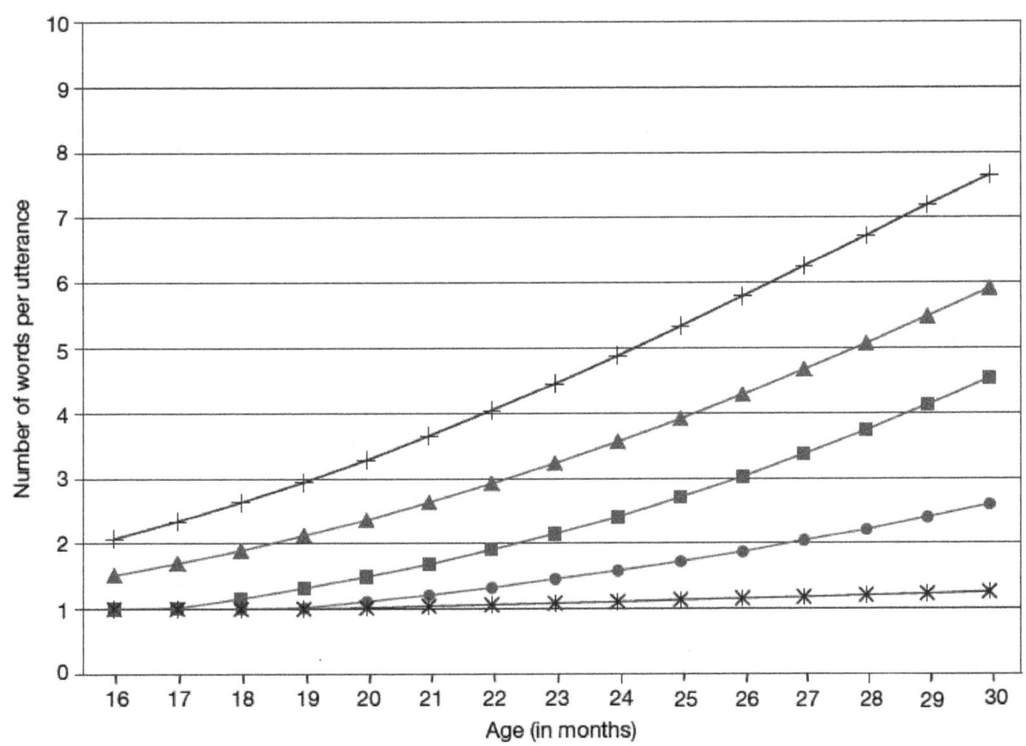

Figure 5.24. *M3L-Palabras* [M3L-*Words] (Inventario II)—boys. (*Key:* —+— 90th percentile; —▲— 75th percentile; —■— 50th percentile; —●—25th percentile; —✳— 10th percentile.)

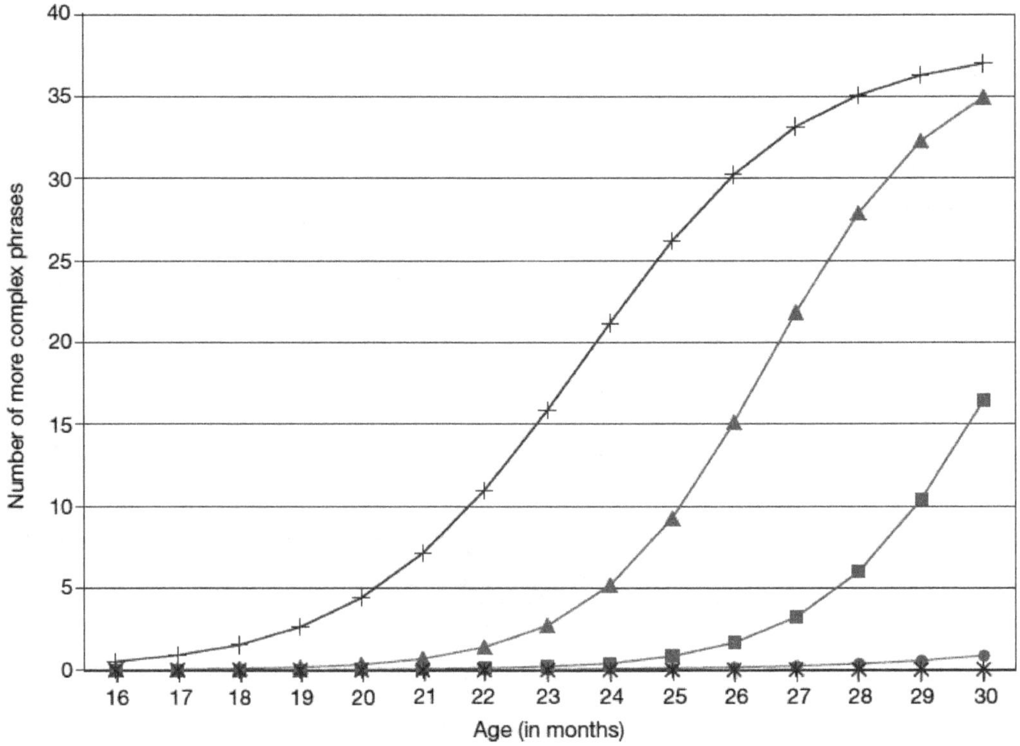

Figure 5.25. *Complejidad de Frases* [Complexity] (Inventario II)—both sexes combined. (*Key:* —+— 90th percentile; —▲— 75th percentile; —■— 50th percentile; —●—25th percentile; —✳— 10th percentile.)

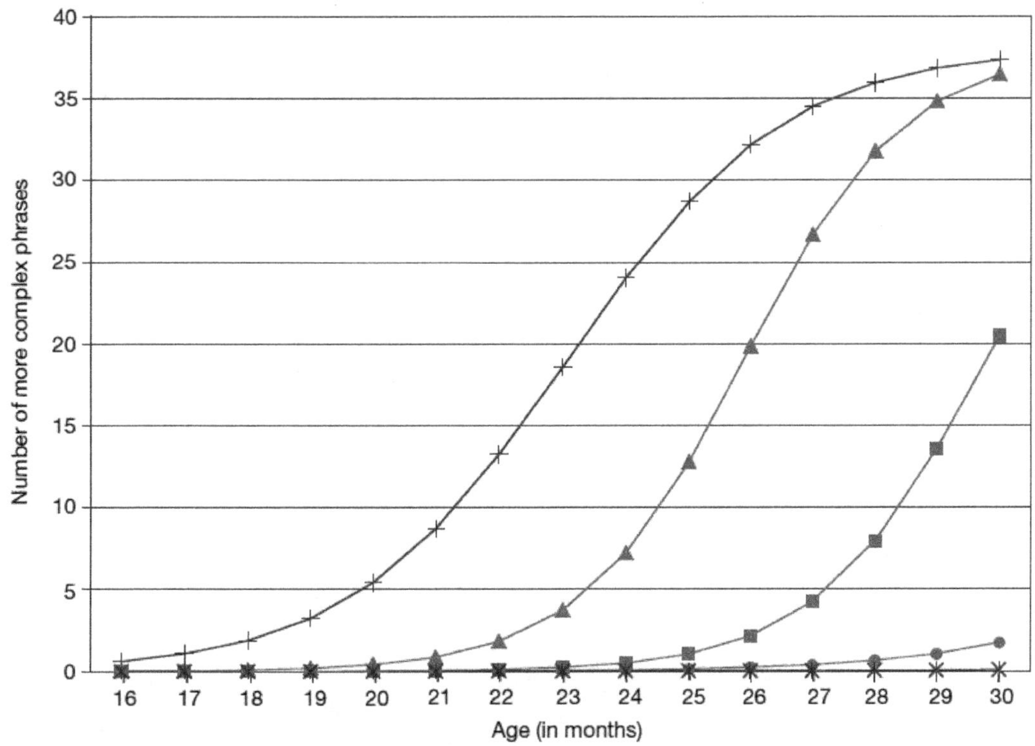

Figure 5.26. *Complejidad de Frases* [Complexity] (Inventario II)—girls. (*Key:* —+— 90th percentile; —▲— 75th percentile; —■— 50th percentile; —●—25th percentile; —✳— 10th percentile.)

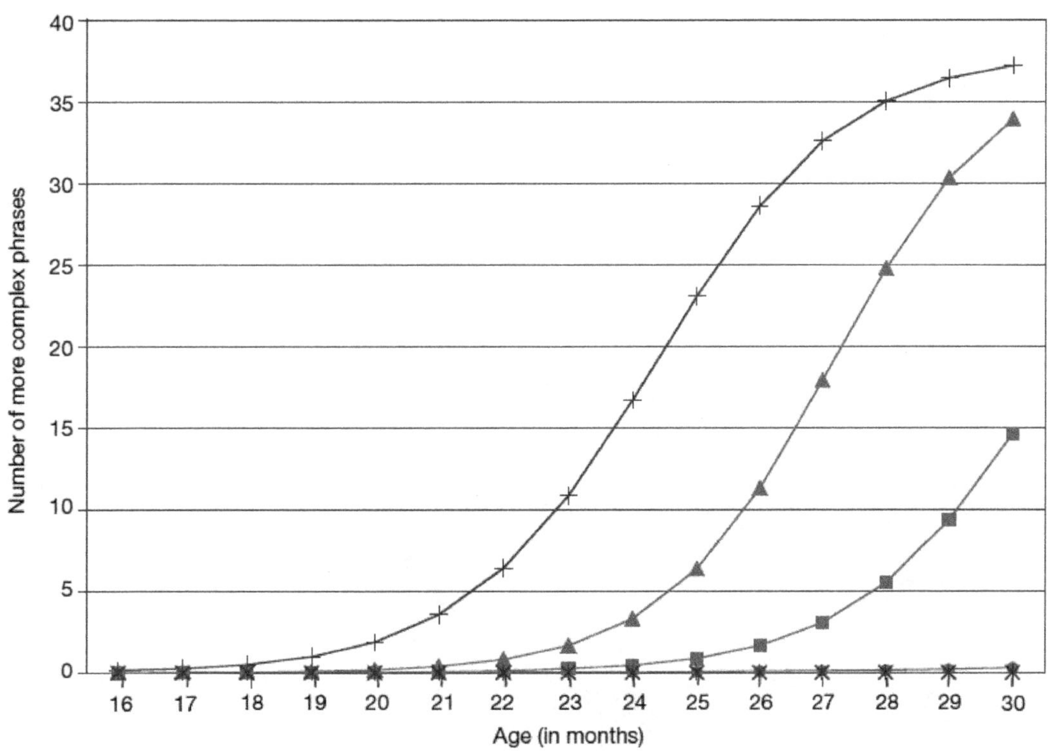

Figure 5.27. *Complejidad de Frases* [Complexity] (Inventario II)—boys. (*Key:* —+— 90th percentile; —▲— 75th percentile; —■— 50th percentile; —●—25th percentile; —✳— 10th percentile.)

REFERENCES

Acredolo, L.P., & Goodwyn, S.W. (1985). Symbolic gesturing in language development: A case study. *Human Development, 28*(1), 40–49.

Acredolo, L.P., & Goodwyn, S.W. (1988). Symbolic gesturing in normal infants. *Child Development, 59*(2), 450–456.

Aguado Alonso, G. (1989). *El desarrollo de la morfosintaxis en el niño.* Madrid, Spain: Ciencias de la Educación Pre-escolar y Especial.

Alarcos Llorach, E. (1976). La adquisición del lenguaje por el niño. In A. Martinez (Ed.), *Tratado de lenguaje* (pp. 9–42). Buenos Aires, Argentina: Nueva Visión.

Anastasi, A. (1988). *Psychological testing* (6th ed.). New York: Macmillan.

Anderson, R. (1995). Spanish morphological and syntactic development. In H. Kayser (Ed.), *Bilingual speech-language pathology: A Hispanic focus* (pp. 41–72). San Diego: Singular Publishing Group.

Arriaga, R.I., Fenson, L., Cronan, T., & Pethick, S. (1998). Scores on the MacArthur Communicative Development Inventory of children from low- and middle-income families. *Applied Psycholinguistics, 19*(2), 209–223.

Bangs, T.E., & Dodson, S. (1979). *Birth to Three Developmental Scale.* Boston: Teaching Resources Corporation.

Bates, E., Beeghly, M., Bretherton, I., McNew, S., Oakes, L., O'Connell, B., Reznick, S., Shore, C., Snyder, L., Volterra, V., & Whitesell, K. (1985). *Language and Gesture Inventory.* Unpublished test materials, University of California, San Diego.

Bates, E., Benigni, L., Bretherton, I., Camaioni, L., & Volterra, V. (1979). *The emergence of symbols: Cognition and communication in infancy.* San Diego: Academic Press.

Bates, E., Bretherton, I., & Snyder, L. (1988). *From first words to grammar: Individual differences and dissociable mechanisms.* New York: Cambridge University Press.

Bates, E., Camaioni, L., & Volterra, V. (1975). The acquisition of performatives prior to speech. *Merrill-Palmer Quarterly, 21*(3), 205–226.

Bates, E., Thal, D., Whitesell, K., Fenson, L., & Oakes, L. (1989). Integrating language and gesture in infancy. *Developmental Psychology, 25*(6), 1004–1019.

Bavin, E. (1992). The acquisition of Walpiri. In D.I. Slobin (Ed.), *The cross-linguistic study of language acquisition* (Vol. 3, pp. 309–371). Mahwah, NJ: Lawrence Erlbaum Associates.

Bayley, N. (1969). *Bayley Scales of Infant Development: Birth to two years.* San Antonio, TX: The Psychological Corporation.

Bayley, N. (1993). *Bayley Scales of Infant Development* (2nd ed.). San Antonio, TX: The Psychological Corporation.

Bedore, L.M. (1999). The acquisition of Spanish. In O.L. Taylor & L.B. Leonard (Eds.), *Language acquisition across North America: Cross-cultural and cross-linguistic perspectives* (pp. 157–208). San Diego: Singular Publishing Group.

Bedore, L.M. (2001). Assessing morphosyntax in Spanish-speaking children. *Seminars in Speech and Language, 22*(1), 65–78.

Beléndez-Soltero, P. (1980). *Repetitions and the acquisition of the Spanish verb system.* Unpublished doctoral dissertation, Harvard University, Cambridge, MA.

Benedict, H. (1979). Early lexical development: Comprehension and production. *Journal of Child Language, 6*(2), 183–200.

Bishop, D.V.M. (1997). *Uncommon understanding: Development and disorders of language comprehension in children.* East Sussex, UK: Psychology Press.

Bloom, L., & Lahey, M. (1978). *Language development and language disorders.* New York: John Wiley & Sons.

Blount, B.G. (1978). Parental speech to children: Cultural patterns. *Language and Language Behavior Abstracts, 12*(3), 2.

Bornstein, M.H., & Haynes, O.M. (1998). Vocabulary competence in early childhood: Measurement, latent construct, and predictive validity. *Child Development, 69*(3), 654–671.

Bornstein, M.H., Haynes, O.M., & Painter, K. (1998). Sources of child vocabulary competence: A multivariate model. *Journal of Child Language, 25*(2), 367–393.

Bornstein, M.H., Tamis-LeMonda, C.S., & Haynes, O.M. (1999). First words in the second year: Continuity, stability, and models of concurrent and predictive correspondence in vocabulary and verbal responsiveness across age and context. *Infant Behavior and Development, 22*(1), 65–85.

Bretherton, I. (1984). Representing the social world in symbolic play: Reality and fantasy. In I. Bretherton (Ed.), *Symbolic play: The development of social understanding.* San Diego: Academic Press.

Brigance, A.H. (1991). *Brigance Inventory of Early Development–Revised.* Billerica, MA: Curriculum Associates, Inc.

Bruner, J. (1977). Early social interactions and language acquisition. In H. Schaffer (Ed.), *Studies in mother-infant interaction.* San Diego: Academic Press.

Burchinal, M., & Appelbaum, M.I. (1991). Estimating individual developmental functions: Methods and their assumptions. *Child Development, 62*(1), 23–43.

Bureau of the Census. (1991). *General population characteristics* (Vol. L). Washington, DC: U.S. Government Printing Office.

Butterworth, G., & Morissette, P. (1996). Onset of pointing and the acquisition of language in infancy. *Journal of Reproductive and Infant Psychology, 14*(3), 219–231.

Bzoch, K.R., & League, R. (1991). *Receptive-Expressive Emergent Language Test–2.* Austin, TX: PRO-ED.

Capirci, O., Iverson, J., Pizzutto, E., & Volterra, V. (1996). Gestures and words during the transition to two-word speech. *Journal of Child Language, 23*(3), 645–673.

Carrillo Aranguren, G., Jackson-Maldonado, D., Thal, D., & Flores, M. (1997). *Language in lower income Spanish-speaking toddlers: Can standard assessment measures be used?* Poster session presented at the Symposium on Research in Child Language Disorders, Madison, WI.

Caselli, M.C. (1990). Communicative gestures and first words. In V. Volterra & C.J. Erting (Eds.), *From gesture to language in hearing and deaf children* (pp. 56–67). New York: Springer-Verlag.

Caselli, M.C., Bates, E., Casadio, P., Fenson, J., Fenson, L., Sanderl, L., & Weir, J. (1995). A cross-linguistic study of early lexical development. *Cognitive Development, 10*(2),159–199.

Caselli, M.C., & Casadio, P. (1992). *Fonzadione MacArthur: Lo sviluppo comunicativo neda prima infanzia.* Rome: Istituto di Psicologia, Consiglio Nazionale delle Ricerche.

Caselli, M.C., & Casadio, P. (1995). *Il primo vocabolario del bambino.* Milan: Franco Angeli.

Conboy, B. (2001, May). *Ties between vocabulary and grammar in simultaneous bilingualism: Implications for emergent literacy.* Paper presented at the fourteenth annual University of California Linguistic Minority Institute conference, Los Angeles.

Conboy, B., & Mills, D. (2001, April). *Two languages, one developing brain: Effects of vocabulary size on bilingual toddlers' event-related potentials to auditory words.* Poster session presented at the biennial meeting of the Society for Research in Child Development, Minneapolis, MN.

Crais, E.R. (1995). Expanding the repertoire of tools and techniques for assessing the communication skills of infants and toddlers. *American Journal of Speech-Language Pathology, 4*(3), 47–59.

Dale, P.S. (1991). The validity of a parent report measure of vocabulary and syntax at 24 months. *Journal of Speech and Hearing Sciences, 34*(3), 565–571.

Dale, P.S. (1996). Parent report assessment of language and communication. In S.F. Warren & J. Reichle (Series Eds.) and K.N. Cole, P.S. Dale, & D.J. Thal (Vol. Eds.), *Communication and language intervention series: Vol. 6. Assessment of communication and language* (pp. 161–182). Baltimore: Paul H. Brookes Publishing Co.

Dale, P.S. (1999). IDHC Score: A scoring program for the Inventario del Desarrollo de Habilidades Comunicativas. Unpublished software.

Dale, P.S., Bates, E., Reznick, S., & Morisset, C. (1989). The validity of a parent report instrument of child language at 20 months. *Journal of Child Language, 16*(2), 239–250.

Dale, P.S., Reznick, S., & Thal, D. (1998). *A parent report measure of language development for three year olds.* Poster session presented at the International Conference on Infant Studies, Atlanta, GA.

Dato, D. (1975). On psycholinguistic universals in children's learning of Spanish. In D. Dato (Ed.), *Developmental psycholinguistics: Theory and applications* (pp. 235–254). Washington, DC: Georgetown University Press.

Delgado-Gaitán, C., & Trueba, T. (1991). *Crossing cultural borders.* New York: Falmer Press.

Demuth, K. (1992). The acquisition of Sesotho. In D.I. Slobin (Ed.), *The cross-linguistic study of language acquisition* (Vol. 3, pp. 557–638). Mahwah, NJ: Lawrence Erlbaum Associates.

Dollaghan, C.A., Campbell, T.F., Paradise, J.L., Feldman, H.M., Jansoky, J.E., Pitcairn, D.N., Kurs-Lasky, M. (1999). Maternal education and measures of early speech and language. *Journal of Speech, Language, and Hearing Research, 42*(6), 1432–1443.

Dromi, E. (1987). *Early lexical development.* New York: Cambridge University Press.

Dunn, L.M., Lugo, D.E., Padilla, E.R., & Dunn, L.M. (1986). *Test de Vocabulario en Imágenes Peabody, Adaptación Hispanoamericana.* Circle Pines, MN: American Guidance Service.

Echeverría, M. (1979). Longitud del enunciado infantil: Factores ambientales e individuales. In *Estudios generales 1: Actas del 5° seminario de investigación y enseñanza de la lingüística* (pp. 56–68). Santiago, Chile: Sociedad Chilena de Lingüística y Universidad Técnica del Estado.

Eisenberg, A. (1985). *Language acquisition in cultural perspective: Talk in three Mexicano homes.* Unpublished doctoral dissertation, University of California, Berkeley.

Farver, J.M. (1993). Cultural differences in scaffolding pretend play. In K. MacDonald (Ed.), *Parent-child play: Descriptions and implications* (pp. 349–366). Albany: SUNY Press.

Feldman, H.M., Dollaghan, C.A., Campbell, T.F., Kurs-Lasky, M., Janosky, J.E., & Paradise, J.L. (2000). Measurement properties of the MacArthur Communicative Development Inventories at ages one and two years. *Child Development, 71*(2), 310–322.

Fenson, L., Bates, E., Dale, P., Goodman, J., Reznick, J.S., & Thal, D. (2000). Measuring variability in early child language: Don't shoot the messenger. *Child Development, 71*(2), 323–328.

Fenson, L., Dale, P.S., Reznick, J.S., Bates, E., Thal, D.J., & Pethick, S.J. (1994). Variability in early communicative development. *Monographs of the Society for Research in Child Development, 59*(5, Serial No. 242).

Fenson, L., Dale, P., Reznick, J.S., Thal, D., Bates, E., Hartung, J.P., Pethick, S., & Reilly, J. (1993). *MacArthur Communicative Development Inventories: User's guide and technical manual.* Baltimore: Paul H. Brookes Publishing Co. (Original copyright assigned 1992)

Fenson, L., Kagan, J., Kearsley, R.B., & Zelazo, P.R. (1976). The developmental progression of manipulative play in the first two years. *Child Development, 47*(1), 232–236.

Fenson, L., Pethick, S., Renda, C., Cox, J.L., Dale, P.S., & Reznick, J.S. (2000). Short-form versions of the MacArthur Communicative Development Inventories. *Applied Psycholinguistics, 21*(1), 95–116.

Fenson, L., & Ramsay, D.S. (1980). Decentration and integration of the child's play in the second year. *Child Development, 51*(1), 171–178.

Fernández Martínez, A.F. (1994). El aprendizaje de los morfemas verbales: Datos de un estudio longitudinal. In S. López Ornat, A. Fernández, P. Gallo, & S. Mariscal (Eds.), *La adquisición de la lengua española* (pp. 29–46). Madrid, Spain: Siglo XXI Editores.

Fischel, J., Whitehurst, G., Caufield, M., & Debaryshe, B. (1989). Language growth in children with expressive language delay. *Pediatrics, 82,* 218–227.

Frankenburg, W.K., Dodds, J.B., Archer, P., Bresnick, B., Maschka, P., Edelman, N., & Shapiro, H. (1992). *Denver II.* Denver, CO: Denver Developmental Materials. (Available from the publisher, Post Office Box 371075, Denver, CO 80327-5075)

García, E. (1978). *Early childhood bilingualism with special reference to the Mexican American child.* Albuquerque: University of New Mexico.

Garcia Coll, C.T. (1990). Developmental outcomes of minority infants: A process-oriented look into our beginnings. *Child Development, 61,* 270–289.

Gardner, M.F. (1981). *Expressive One-Word Picture Vocabulary Test.* Novato, CA: Academic Therapy Publications.

Gardner, M.F. (1990). *Expressive One-Word Picture Vocabulary Test–Revised* (Spanish version). Novato, CA: Academic Therapy Publications.

Gathercole, V.M., Sebastián, E., & Soto, P. (1999). The early acquisition of Spanish verbal morphology: Across-the-board or piecemeal knowledge? *International Journal of Bilingualism, 2,* 72–89.

Girolametto, L., Pearce, P.S., & Weitzman, E. (1996). Interactive focused stimulation for toddlers with expressive vocabulary delays. *Journal of Speech and Hearing Research, 39*(6), 1274–1283.

Girolametto, L., Pearce, P.S., & Weitzman, E. (1997). Effects of lexical intervention on the phonology of late talkers. *Journal of Speech, Language, and Hearing Research, 40*(2), 338–348.

Girolametto, L., Weitzman, E., Wiigs, M., & Pearce, P.S. (1999). The relationship between maternal language measures and language development in toddlers with expressive vocabulary delays. *American Journal of Speech-Language Pathology, 8*(4), 364–374.

Goldin-Meadow, S., & Morford, M. (1985). Gesture in early child language: Studies of deaf and hearing children. *Merrill-Palmer Quarterly, 31*(2), 145–176.

Gómez Palacio, M. (1988). *Batería de Evaluación de la Lengua Española.* Mexico City, Mexico: Dirección General de Educación Especial.

Gómez Palacio, M., Padilla, E., & Roll, S. (1982). *WISC-RM: Wechsler Intelligence Scale for Children–Revised (Mexicano).* Mexico City, Mexico: Editorial el Manual Moderno.

González, G. (1983). Expressing time through verb tenses and temporal expressions in Spanish: Age 2.0–4.6. *NABE Journal, 7*(2), 69–82.

Gutiérrez, L. (1976). *A study of the applicability of Halliday's functional theory of language development to two Spanish-speaking children at the pre-syntactic stage.* Unpublished doctoral dissertation, University of New Mexico, Albuquerque.

Gutierrez-Clellen, V.F. (1996). Language diversity: Implications for assessment. In S.F. Warren & J. Reichle (Series Eds.) and K.N. Cole, P.S. Dale, & D.J. Thal (Vol. Eds.), *Communication and language intervention series, Vol. 6. Assessment of communication and language* (pp. 29–56). Baltimore: Paul H. Brookes Publishing Co.

Gutiérrez-Clellen, V.F., Restrepo, M.A., Bedore, L., Peña, E., & Anderson, R. (2000). Language sample analysis in Spanish-speaking children: Methodological considerations. *Language, Speech, and Hearing Services in Schools, 31,* 88–98.

Hart, B., & Risley, T.R. (1995). *Meaningful differences in the everyday experience of young American children.* Baltimore: Paul H. Brookes Publishing Co.

Heath, S.B. (1983). *Ways with words: Language, life and work in communities and classrooms.* New York: Cambridge University Press.

Heath, S.B. (1986). Sociocultural contexts of language development. In *Beyond language: Social and cultural factors in schooling language minority children* (pp. 143–186). Los Angeles: California State University, Evaluation Dissemination and Assessment Center.

Hedrick, D.L., Prather, E.M., & Tobin, A.R. (1984). *Sequenced Inventory of Communication Development–Revised Edition (SICD-R).* Seattle: University of Washington Press.

Hedrick, D.L., Prather, E.M., & Tobin, A.R. (1984). *Sequenced Inventory of Communicative Development–Spanish Translation* (L. Rosenberg, Trans.). Seattle: University of Washington Press.

Hernández Pina, F. (1984). *Teorías psico-sociolingüísticas y su aplicación a la adquisición del español como lengua materna.* Madrid, Spain: Siglo XXI Editores.

Huebner, C.E. (2000). Community-based support for preschool readiness among children in poverty. *Journal of Education for Students Placed at Risk, 5*(3), 291–314.

Iglesias, A. (1985). Communication in the home and classroom: Match or mismatch? *Topics in Language Disorders, 5*(4), 29–41.

Individuals with Disabilities Education Act Amendments of 1997, PL 105-17, 20 U.S.C. §§ 1400 *et seq.*

Instituto Nacional de Estadística, Geografía e Informática. (1997). *Censo General de Población y Vivienda.* Mexico City, Mexico: Author.

Iverson, J., Capirci, O., & Caselli, M.C. (1994). From communication to language in two modalities. *Cognitive Development, 9*(1), 23–43.

Jackson, D. (1989). *Una palabra: Multiplicidad de intenciones y funciones.* Unpublished doctoral dissertation, El Colegio de Mexico, Mexico City, Mexico.

Jackson, S.C. (1996). *Family and professional congruence in communication assessments of preschool boys with Fragile X syndrome (mental retardation).* Unpublished doctoral dissertation, University of North Carolina at Chapel Hill.

Jackson-Maldonado, D. (1984). Unpublished child language transcripts.

Jackson-Maldonado, D. (1988). Evaluación del lenguaje infantil: Enfoque transcultural. In A. Ardila & F. Ostrosky-Solis (Eds.), *Lenguaje oral y escrito* (pp. 92–118). Mexico City, Mexico: Editores Trillas.

Jackson-Maldonado, D. (1994). *Lenguaje y Cognición en los Primeros Años de Vida: Fase 2.* Project financed by the Consejo Nacional de Ciencia y Tecnología (CONACYT), Mexico City, Mexico.

Jackson-Maldonado, D. (1997). *Early communicative abilities of Spanish-speaking children: Vocabulary, phrases and gestures.* Seminar presented at the Research Symposium on Language Diversity in Multicultural Communication Sciences and Disorders, Austin, TX.

Jackson-Maldonado, D. (1999). Early language assessment for Spanish-speaking children: Border realities. In T. Fletcher & C. Bos (Eds.), *Social integration of children with disabilities and their families: Blending U.S. and Mexican perspectives* (pp. 35–52). Tempe, AZ: Bilingual Press.

Jackson-Maldonado, D. (2000). *Spanish verbal morphology acquisition.* Symposium on Clinical Linguistic Studies of Spanish Speakers: Child Language. Annual convention of the American Speech-Language-Hearing Association, Washington, DC.

Jackson-Maldonado, D., & Maldonado, R. (2001). Determinaciones semánticas de la flexión verbal en la adquisición del español. In C. Rojas-Nieto & L. de León (Eds.), *Estudios de Adquisición del Lenguaje Español y Lenguas Indígenas* (pp. 165–200). Mexico City, Mexico: UNAM-IIFL-CIESAS.

Jackson-Maldonado, D., Thal, D., Marchman, V., Bates, E., & Gutierrez-Clellen, V. (1993). Early lexical development of Spanish-speaking infants and toddlers. *Journal of Child Language, 20*(3), 523–549.

Kayser, H. (1995). Assessment of speech and language impairments in bilingual children. In H. Kayser (Ed.), *Bilingual speech-language pathology: A Hispanic focus* (pp. 243–263). San Diego: Singular Press.

Kaufman, A., Kaufman, N., Gómez Palacio, M., Rangel, E., & Padilla, E. (1987). *Batería de Evaluación Intelectual Kaufman.* Mexico City, Mexico: Dirección General de Educación Especial.

Keppel, G. (1991). *Design and analysis: A researcher's handbook* (3rd ed.). Upper Saddle River, NJ: Prentice-Hall.

Klee, T., Carson, D., Gavin, W., Hall, L., Kent, A., & Reece, S. (1998). Concurrent and predictive validity of an early language screening program. *Journal of Speech, Language, and Hearing Research, 41,* 627–641.

Klee, T., Pearce, K., & Carson, D. (2000). Improving the positive predictive value of screening for developmental language disorder. *Journal of Speech, Language, and Hearing Disorders, 43,* 821–833.

Kvaal, J.T., Shipstead-Cox, N., Nevitt, S., Hodson, B., & Launer, P. (1988). The acquisition of 10 Spanish morphemes by Spanish-speaking children. *Language, Speech, and Hearing Services in Schools, 19,* 384–394.

Laakso, M.-L., Poikkeus, A.-M., Eklund, K., & Lyytinen, P. (1999). Social interactional behaviors and symbolic play competence as predictors of language development and their associations with maternal attention-directing strategies. *Infant Behavior and Development, 22*(4), 541–556.

Lahey, M. (1988). *Language disorders and language development.* New York: Macmillan.

Langdon, H.W. (1992a). Language communication and sociocultural patterns in Hispanic families. In H.W. Langdon & L.L. Cheng (Ed.), *Hispanic children and adults with communication disorders: Assessment and intervention* (pp. 99–131). Gaithersburg, MD: Aspen Publishers.

Langdon, H.W. (1992b). Speech and language assessment of LEP/bilingual Hispanic students. In H.W. Langdon & L.L. Cheng (Ed.), *Hispanic children and adults with communication disorders: Assessment and intervention* (pp. 201–271). Gaithersburg, MD: Aspen Publishers.

Laosa, L. (1982). School, occupation, culture, and family: The impact of parental schooling on the parent–child relationship. *Journal of Educational Psychology, 74*(6), 791–827.

Lawrence, C.W. (1992). Assessing the use of age-equivalent scores in clinical management. *Language, Speech, and Hearing Services in Schools, 23*(1), 6–8.

Leonard, L.B. (1998). *Children with specific language impairment.* Cambridge, MA: The MIT Press.

Leopold, W.F. (1949). *Speech development of a bilingual child: A linguist's record* (Vol. 3). Evanston, IL: Northwestern University Press.

Linares-Orama, N., & Sanders, L.J. (1977). Evaluation of syntax in three-year-old Spanish-speaking Puerto Rican children. *Journal of Speech and Hearing Research, 20,* 350–357.

Locke, A. (1978). *Action, gesture, and symbol.* San Diego: Academic Press.

López Ornat, S. (1988). On data sources on the acquisition of Spanish as a first language. *Journal of Child Language, 15*(3), 679–688.

López Ornat, S., Fernández, A., Gallo, P., & Mariscal, S. (1994). *La adquisición de la lengua española.* Madrid, Spain: Siglo XXI Editores.

Lund, N.J., & Duchan, J.F. (1988). *Assessing children's language in naturalistic contexts* (2nd ed.). Upper Saddle River, NJ: Prentice-Hall.

Lyytinen, P., Poikkeus, A.M., Leiwo, M., Ahonen, T., & Lyytinen, H. (1996). Parents as informants of their child's vocal and early language development. *Early Child Development and Care, 126,* 15–25.

Maez, L. (1983). The acquisition of noun and verb morphology in 18–24 month-old Spanish speaking children. *NABE Journal, 7,* 53–68.

Marchman, V.A., & Martínez-Sussmann, C. (2002). Concurrent validity of caregiver/parent report measures of language for children who are learning both English and Spanish. *Journal of Speech, Language, and Hearing Research, 45*(5), 993–997.

Mattes, L.J., & Omark, D.R. (1991). *Speech and language assessment for the bilingual handicapped* (2nd ed.). Oceanside, CA: Academic Communication Associates.

Merino, B.J., Figueroa, R.A., Gómez Palacio, M., Rangel Hinojosa, E., & Jackson-Maldonado, D. (1987). *Sistema de Evaluación Sobre la Adquisición de la Lengua Española (SEALE).* Mexico City, Mexico: Oficina de Educación Especial, Secretaría de Educación Pública.

Merino, B., & Spencer, M. (1983). The comparability of English and Spanish versions of oral language proficiency instruments. *NABE Journal, 7,* 1–31.

Miller, J.F. (1981). *Assessing language production in children: Experimental procedures.* Baltimore: University Park Press.

Miller, J.F., Sedey, A.L., & Miolo, G. (1995). Validity of parent report measures of vocabulary development for children with Down syndrome. *Journal of Speech and Hearing Research, 38,* 1037–1044.

Ochs, E. (1982). Talking to children in Western Samoa. *Language Socialization, 11*(1), 77–104.

Patterson, J. (1998). Expressive vocabulary development and word combinations of Spanish-English bilingual toddlers. *American Journal of Speech-Language Pathology, 7*(4), 46–56.

Patterson, J. (2000). Observed and reported expressive vocabulary and word combinations in bilingual toddlers. *Journal of Speech, Language, and Hearing Research, 43*(1), 121–128.

Paul, R. (1996). Clinical implications of the natural history of slow expressive language development. *American Journal of Speech-Language Pathology, 5*(2), 5–21.

Paul, R. (1997). Understanding language delay: A reply to van Kleeck, Gillam, and Davis. *American Journal of Speech-Language Pathology, 6*(2), 40–49.

Pearson, B.Z., Fernandez, S., & Oller, D.K. (1995a). Cross-language synonyms in the lexicons of bilingual infants: One language or two? *Journal of Child Language, 22,* 345–368.

Pearson, B.Z., Fernandez, S., & Oller, D.K. (1995b). Lexical development in bilingual infants and toddlers: Comparison to monolingual norms. In B. Harley (Ed.). (1995). *Lexical issues in language learning* (pp. 31–57). Toronto: OISE. (Reprinted from *Language Learning, 43*[1; 1993], 93–120.)

Pérez, M., & Castro, J. (1988). Fenómenos transicionales en el acceso al lenguaje. *Infancia y aprendizaje, 43,* 13–36.

Piaget, J. (1952). *The origins of intelligence in children.* New York: International Universities Press.

Piaget, J. (1962). *Play, dreams, and imitation in childhood.* New York: W.W. Norton.

Rescorla, L. (1989). The Language Development Survey: A screening tool for delayed language in toddlers. *Journal of Speech and Hearing Disorders, 54*(4), 587–599.

Rescorla, L. (1991). Identifying expressive language delay at age two. *Topics in Language Disorders, 11*(4), 14–20.

Rescorla, L. (2000). Do late-talking toddlers turn out to have reading difficulties a decade later? *Annals of Dyslexia, 50,* 87–102.

Rescorla, L., & Alley, A. (2001). Validation of the Language Development Survey (LDS): A parent report tool for identifying language delay in toddlers. *Journal of Speech, Language, and Hearing Research, 44*(2), 434–445.

Rescorla, L., & Schwartz, E. (1990). Outcome of toddlers with specific expressive language delay. *Applied Psycholinguistics, 11*(4), 393–407.

Reznick, J.S. (1990). Visual preference as a test of infant word comprehension. *Applied Psycholinguistics, 11,* 145–166.

Roberts, J.E., Burchinal, M., & Durham, M. (1999). Parents' report of vocabulary and grammatical development of African American preschoolers: Child and environmental associations. *Child Development, 70*(1), 92–106.

Robertson, S.B., & Weismer, S.E. (1999). Effects of treatment on linguistic and social skills in toddlers with delayed language development. *Journal of Speech, Language, and Hearing Research, 42*(5), 1234–1248.

Rollins, P.R., & Snow, C.E. (1998). Shared attention and grammatical development in typical children and children with autism. *Journal of Child Language, 25*(3), 653–673.

Roopnarine, J., Johnson, J., & Hooper, F. (Eds.). (1994). *Children's play in diverse cultures.* Albany: SUNY Press.

Rossetti, L. (1995). *The Rossetti Infant-Toddler Language Scale: A Measure of Communication and Interaction.* East Moline, IL: LinguiSystems.

Sattler, J. M. (1988). *Assessment of children* (3rd ed.). San Diego: Singular Publishing Group.

Saxon, T.F. (1997). A longitudinal study of early mother–infant interaction and later language competence. *First Language, 17,* 271–281.

Scherer, N.J. (1999). The speech and language status of toddlers with cleft lip and/or palate following early vocabulary intervention. *American Journal of Speech-Language Pathology, 8*(1), 81–93.

Schieffelin, B., & Eisenberg, A. (1984). Cultural variation in children's conversations. In R.L. Schiefelbusch & J. Pickar (Eds.), *The acquisition of communicative competence.* Baltimore: University Park Press.

Schieffelin, B., & Ochs, E. (1986). *Language socialization across cultures.* New York: Cambridge University Press.

Schnell de Acedo, B. (1994). Early morphological development: The acquisition of articles in Spanish. In J.L. Sokolov & C. Snow (Eds.), *Handbook of research in language development using CHILDES* (pp. 210–253). Mahwah, NJ: Lawrence Erlbaum Associates.

Slobin, D.I. (Ed.). (1985). *The cross-linguistic study of language acquisition* (Vols. 1 & 2). Mahwah, NJ: Lawrence Erlbaum Associates.

Snyder, L., Bates, E., & Bretherton, I. (1981). Content and context in early language development. *Journal of Child Language, 8*(3), 565–582.

Stern, C., & Stern, W. (1907). *Die kindersprache: Eine psychologische und sprachtheoretische Untersuchung.* Leipzig, Germany: Berth.

Tamis-LeMonda, C., & Bornstein, M. (1990). Language, play, and attention at one year. *Infant Behavior and Development, 13*(1), 85–98.

Terrell, B., & Schwartz, R. (1988). Object transformations in the play of language-impaired children. *Journal of Speech and Hearing Disorders, 53*(4), 459–466.

Terrell, B., Schwartz, R., Prelock, P., & Messick, C. (1984). Symbolic play in normal and language impaired children. *Journal of Speech and Hearing Research, 27*(3), 424–429.

Thal, D. (2000). *Late-talking toddlers: Are they at risk?* San Diego: San Diego State University Press.

Thal, D., & Bates, E. (1988). Language and gesture in late talkers. *Journal of Speech and Hearing Research, 31*(1), 115–123.

Thal, D.J., Bates, E., Zappia, M.J., & Oroz, M. (1996). Ties between lexical and grammatical development: Evidence from early-talkers. *Journal of Child Language, 23*(2), 349–368.

Thal, D., Jackson-Maldonado, D., & Acosta, D. (2000). Validity of a parent report measure of vocabulary and grammar for Spanish-speaking toddlers. *Journal of Speech, Language, and Hearing Research, 43,* 1087–1100.

Thal, D., Jackson-Maldonado, D., & Fenson, L. (1999, July). *Fundación MacArthur: Inventario del Desarrollo de Habilidades Comunicativas—Norms and validation studies.* Poster session presented at the eighth International Conference for the Study of Child Language, San Sebastián, Spain.

Thal, D.J., & Katich, J. (1996). Predicaments in early identification of specific language impairment: Does the early bird always catch the worm? In S.F. Warren & J. Reichle (Series Eds.) and K.N. Cole, P.S. Dale, & D.J. Thal (Vol. Eds.), *Communication and language intervention series: Vol. 6. Assessment of communication and language* (pp. 1–28). Baltimore: Paul H. Brookes Publishing Co.

Thal, D.J., O'Hanlon, L., Clemmons, M., & Fralin, L. (1999). Validity of a parent report measure of vocabulary and syntax for preschool children with language impairment. *Journal of Speech, Language, and Hearing Research, 42*(2), 482–496.

Thal, D., & Tobias, S. (1992). Communicative gestures in children with delayed onset of oral expressive vocabulary. *Journal of Speech and Hearing Research, 35*(6), 1281–1289.

Thal, D., & Tobias, S. (1994). Relationships between language and gesture in normal developing and late-talking toddlers. *Journal of Speech and Hearing Research, 37*(1), 157–170.

Thal, D., Tobias, S., & Morrison, D. (1991). Language and gesture in late talkers: A one year follow-up. *Journal of Speech and Hearing Research, 34*(3), 604–612.

Tomasello, M. (1992). *First verbs: A case study of early grammatical development.* New York: Cambridge University Press.

Tomasello, M., & Farrar, J. (1986). Joint attention and early language. *Child Development, 57,* 1454–1463.

Tomasello, M., & Mervis, C.B. (1994). The instrument is great, but measuring comprehension is still a problem. In L. Fenson, P. Dale, J.S. Reznick, E. Bates, D. Thal, & S. Pethick, Variability in early communicative development. *Monographs of the Society for Research in Child Development, 59*(5, Serial No. 242), 174–179.

Truex, N.W. (1982). *An interactive concept of language development with reference to Spanish.* Unpublished doctoral dissertation, University of California, Los Angeles.

Umbel, V.M., Pearson, B.Z., Fernandez, M.C., & Oller, D.K. (1992). Measuring bilingual children's receptive vocabularies. *Child Development, 63,* 1012–1020.

van Kleeck, A., & Richardson, A. (1990). Assessment of speech and language development. In J.H. Johnson & J. Goldman (Eds.), *Developmental assessment in clinical child psychology* (pp. 132–172). New York: Pergamon Press.

Walker, D., Greenwood, C., Hart, B., & Carta, J. (1994). Prediction of school outcomes based on early language production and socioeconomic factors. *Child Development, 65,* 606–621.

Willis, S., & Edwards, J. (1996). A prelingually deaf child's acquisition of spoken vocabulary in the first year of multichannel cochlear implant use. *Child Language Teaching and Therapy, 12*(3), 272–287.

Yoder, P.J., Warren, S.F., & Biggar, H.A. (1997). Stability of maternal reports of lexical comprehension in very young children with developmental delays. *American Journal of Speech-Language Pathology, 6*(1), 59–64.

Yoder, P.J., Warren, S.F., & McCathren, R.B. (1998). Determining spoken language prognosis in children with developmental disabilities. *American Journal of Speech-Language Pathology, 7*(4), 77–87.

Zimmerman, I.L., Steiner, V.G., & Pond, R.E. (1993a). *Preschool Language Scale–3.* San Antonio, TX: The Psychological Corporation.

Zimmerman, I.L., Steiner, V.G., & Pond, R.E. (1993b). *Preschool Language Scale–3, Spanish Edition.* San Antonio, TX: The Psychological Corporation.

Zukow, P.G. (1984). Folk theories of comprehension and caregiver style in a rural-born population in Central Mexico. *Quarterly Newsletter of the Laboratory of Comparative Human Cognition, 6,* 62–67.

Zukow-Goldring, P. (2001). Perceiving referring actions: Latino and Euro-American infants and caregivers comprehending speech. In K.E. Nelson, A. Aksu-Koç, & C.E. Johnson (Eds.), *Children's language series: Vol. 11. Interactional contributions to language development.* Mahwah, NJ: Lawrence Erlbaum Associates.

A

BASIC INFORMATION FORM/ *FORMA DE INFORMACIÓN BÁSICA*

Basic Information Form

ID number ______________ Today's date __________________ Child's birth date ___________________

Child's name ____ Gender _________

FIRST MIDDLE LAST

Address ____ Telephone (___)___________

STREET CITY STATE ZIP

Child's birth order ☐ 1st ☐ 2nd ☐ Other (specify) _________ Number of children in family _____

Is child adopted? ☐ yes ☐ no Child's birth weight ____________

Name of mother/guardian ____

FIRST LAST

Name of father/guardian ____

FIRST LAST

HEALTH

Did you experience any major *pregnancy or birth complications?* ☐ yes ☐ no

If yes, please describe ____

Was your child born prematurely (i.e., before the due date)? ☐ yes ☐ no

If yes, how many weeks early? __________

Does your child experience *chronic ear infections* (5 or more)? ☐ yes ☐ no

If yes, has your child undergone intervention (e.g., tube insertion)? ☐ yes ☐ no

If yes, please describe ____

Is there some reason to suspect that your child may have a *hearing loss?* ☐ yes ☐ no

Has your child had any *major illnesses, hospitalizations, or diagnosed disabilities?* ☐ yes ☐ no

If yes, please describe ____

Have *you or any member of your extended family* (e.g., child's siblings, grandmother, father, etc.) been diagnosed with any behavioral impairment, neurological impairment, language or learning disability? ☐ yes ☐ no

If yes, please describe ____

Do you have *any concerns about your child's speech and/or language?* ☐ yes ☐ no

If yes, please describe ____

EXPOSURE TO OTHER LANGUAGES

Is your child *regularly exposed to a language(s) other than English?* ☐ yes ☐ no

If yes: What language(s)? ______________________ By whom? ______________________

Number of days per week? _____ Number of hours per day? ______ Since what age (in months)? _______

Basic Information Form *(continued)*

CAREGIVER INFORMATION

With whom does your child live?

☐ One parent ☐ Both biological parents ☐ Biological parent and stepparent

☐ Adoptive parent(s) ☐ Other, please explain ______________________________

Who participates in the day-to-day care of your child?
(Check all that apply.)

☐ Mother/guardian ☐ Day care center (_________ hrs/week)

☐ Father/guardian ☐ Non-parent caregiver (e.g., grandparent, "nanny") in *your* home (_________ hrs/week)

☐ Outside-the-home caregiver (e.g., "family provider" in that person's home) (_________ hrs/week)

☐ Other, please explain ______________________________ (_________ hrs/week)

ETHNIC BACKGROUND

Please specify your ethnic background (e.g., Asian, Black, Caucasian, Hispanic, Native American, other ethnic group).

______________________________ ______________________________
Mother/guardian Father/guardian

EDUCATION

Please circle the highest grade completed
(12 = high school graduate, 16 = college graduate, 18 = advanced degree).

Mother/guardian: 0 1 2 3 4 5 6 7 8 9 10 11 12 13 14 15 16 17 18

Father/guardian: 0 1 2 3 4 5 6 7 8 9 10 11 12 13 14 15 16 17 18

OCCUPATION

Please provide a brief description of your *occupation* using specific terms
(e.g., computer technician, accountant, dental assistant).

Mother/guardian ______________________________

Father/guardian ______________________________

Approximate annual family income ($) ______________

CONTACT INFORMATION

Name of parent or guardian competing this form ______________________________

The best *time* to contact me is ______________________________

The best *place* to contact me is ☐ Home Telephone ______________

☐ Work Telephone ______________

Thank you for taking the time to answer our questions!
Please contact us if you have any questions or concerns.

Forma de Información Básica

MacArthur INVENTARIOS

Número de identificación _____ Fecha de hoy ___________ Fecha de nacimiento del niño/a ___________

Nombre del niño/a ____ Sexo __________
NOMBRE APELLIDO

Dirección ____ Teléfono (___) __________
CALLE CIUDAD ESTADO CÓDIGO POSTAL

Orden de nacimiento ☐ 1º ☐ 2º ☐ Otro (especifique) _________ Número de niños en la familia _____

¿El niño/a es adoptado? ☐ sí ☐ no Peso del niño/a al nacer ______________

Nombre de la madre/custodio legal ____
NOMBRE APELLIDO

Nombre del padre/custodio legal ____
NOMBRE APELLIDO

SALUD

¿Tuvo usted complicaciones mayores *durante el embarazo o el parto?* ☐ sí ☐ no

En caso positivo, por favor describa ____

¿Su hijo/a fue *prematuro?* (nació antes de la fecha probable del parto) ☐ sí ☐ no

En caso positivo, por favor describa ____

¿Padece su niño/a *de infecciones crónicas del oído* (5 ó mas al año)? ☐ sí ☐ no

¿En este caso, ha recibido su hijo/a algún tipo de intervención médica? ☐ sí ☐ no

En caso positivo, por favor describa ____

¿Sospecha que su niño/a haya sufrido *pérdida en su capacidad auditiva?* ☐ sí ☐ no

En caso positivo, por favor describa ____

¿Su hijo/a ha tenido *enfermedades serias, hospitalizaciones o ha sido diagnostica do con alguna incapacidad?* ☐ sí ☐ no

En caso positivo, por favor describa ____

¿Algún miembro de *su familia (ej., hijos, abuelos, padres, etc.) o usted ha sido diagnosticado con algún tipo de problema de conducta, neurológico, del lenguaje o de aprendizaje?* ☐ sí ☐ no

En caso positivo, por favor especifique ____

¿Alguna vez le ha *preocupado algo sobre el desarrollo del lenguaje* de su hijo? ☐ sí ☐ no

En caso positivo, por favor especifique ____

CONTACTO CON OTRAS LENGUAS

¿El niño/a *tiene contacto regularmente con el español?* ☐ sí ☐ no

En caso positivo: ¿Con quién? ______________________ Número de días por semana _________

Número de horas por día ______ Desde que edad _______ (en meses)

¿El niño/a *tiene contacto regularmente con el inglés?* ☐ sí ☐ no

En caso positivo: ¿Con quién? ______________________ Número de días por semana _________

Número de horas por día ______ Desde que edad _______ (en meses)

¿El niño/a *tiene contacto con otras lenguas aparte del inglés y español?* ☐ sí ☐ no

En caso positivo: ¿Cuál(es) lengua(s)? ________________ ¿Con quién? ________________

Número de días por semana ______ Número de horas por día ______ Desde que edad _____ (en meses)

Forma de Información Básica *(página 2)*

INFORMACION SOBRE EL CUIDADO DEL NIÑO/A

¿Con quién vive el niño/a?

☐ Un padre ☐ Los dos padres biológicos ☐ Padre biológico + padrastro/madrastra

☐ Padres adoptivo(s) ☐ Otro, por favor explique ______________________________

¿Quién participa en el cuidado diario de su niño/a?
(Marque *todo* lo aplicable.)

☐ Madre/custodio legal ☐ Padre/custodio legal ☐ Guardería (________ horas/semana)

☐ Persona que lo/a cuida (ej., abuelos, niñera) en *su* casa (________ horas/semana)

☐ Persona que lo/a cuida *en una casa particular* (________ horas/semana)

☐ Otro, por favor explique ______________________________ (________ horas/semana)

INFORMACIÓN ÉTNICA

Por favor especifique a qué grupo pertenence de los que están enumerados a continuacíon
(ej., afro-americano/a, asiático/a, blanco/a, hispano/a, indígena, indígena americano, u otra categoría).

______________________________ ______________________________

Madre/custodio legal Padre/custodio legal

EDUCACIÓN

Marque el *nivel más alto de estudios* que haya completado
(12 = graduado de nivel medio superior, 16 = graduado universitario, 18 = Maestría ó Doctorado).

Madre/custodio legal: 1 2 3 4 5 6 7 8 9 10 11 12 13 14 15 16 17 18

Padre/custodio legal: 1 2 3 4 5 6 7 8 9 10 11 12 13 14 15 16 17 18

OCUPACIÓN

Por favor, proporcione una descripción breve de su ocupación usando términos específicos
(ej., técnico en computación, asistente dental, maestra, mecánico, etc.)

Madre/custodio legal ______________________________

Padre/custodio legal ______________________________

Salario anual familiar ________________

INFORMACIÓN PARA PONERNOS EN CONTACTO CON USTED

Nombre del padre o custodio legal que llenó esta forma ______________________________

¿Podríamos contactarlo/la para hacerle más preguntas
o para aclarar algunas dudas acerca de esta forma? ☐ sí ☐ no

La mejor *hora* para contactarme es ______________________________

El mejor *lugar* para contactarme es ☐ En casa Teléfono ________________

☐ En el trabajo Teléfono ________________

Gracias por tomarse el tiempo en contestar este cuestionario.
Si tiene alguna pregunta o duda, favor de contactar al coordinador.

B

GENERAL INSTRUCTIONS/ *INSTRUCCIONES GENERALES*

MacArthur INVENTARIOS

INSTRUCTIONS FOR FILLING OUT THE LANGUAGE QUESTIONNAIRE

A Few Things to Remember

Indicate ***date of birth*** and ***today's date*** on form.

Complete the ***Basic Information Form.***

Please ***read instructions*** carefully!

Make sure you ***complete all of the pages*** of the questionnaire.

For Inventario I, mark the words that your child ***comprende* [understands]** or ***comprende y dice* [understands and says].** For Inventario II, mark the words that your child ***comprende y dice* [understands and says].**

Do not mark ***imitations.***

Give your child ***credit for mispronounced or child words*** (e.g., "pato" for "zapato").

Mark ***words with the same meaning*** as what your child understands or says (e.g., "super" for "tienda").

Take into account ***names of people*** (e.g., "tita" for "abuela") or ***words that are specific to your dialect/region.***

Take into account ***other verb forms*** (e.g., mark "dormir" if your child says "duerme").

Ask others (e.g., other family members, nanny, child care providers) to help you fill out this form.

Thank you very much!

MacArthur INVENTARIOS

INSTRUCCIONES PARA LLENAR EL INVENTARIO

Recuerde

Anote ***la fecha de nacimiento*** y ***la fecha de hoy.***

Llene toda la información en la ***Forma de Informacíon Básica.***

Por favor, lea ***todas las instrucciones*** con cuidado.

Asegúrese de llenar ***todas las páginas*** del inventario.

En el Inventario I, anote las palabras que su hijo/a ***comprende*** o ***comprende y dice.*** En el Inventario II, anote las palabras que su hijo/a ***comprende y dice.***

No indique palabras que sean ***imitaciones.***

Indique ***las palabras aunque el niño/a no las pronuncie bien o sean palabras "infantiles"*** (ej., "pato" en vez de "zapato").

Indique ***las palabras que sean diferentes,*** pero que tienen el mismo significado que las que vienen en la forma (ej., "super" en vez de "tienda").

Tome en cuenta ***los nombres de las personas*** (ej., "tita" en vez de "abuela" o "Juan" en vez de "tío") o palabras que sean de su ***region o dialecto.***

Marque ***formas distintas de los verbos*** (ej., para "dormir", el niño/a puede decir "duerme").

Consulte ***a otras personas*** que tienen contacto con el niño/a (ej., en la guardería, la nana, la abuela).

¡Muchas gracias!

C

FURTHER INSTRUCTIONS AND EXAMPLES

When parents are filling out the *Lista de Vocabulario* [Vocabulary Checklist] of Inventario I and II, it may be helpful to remind them that they should give their child credit for *comprende y dice* [understands and says] even if the child does not pronounce the word perfectly. For example, parents should mark words that the child uses consistently even if the child uses a childlike version of the word (e.g., *pato* instead of *zapato*). In addition, instead of the word on *Lista de Vocabulario* [Vocabulary Checklist], a child may use a different word that has the same meaning. Children sometimes have their own "special" words for things or people in their family. These words may be particular to the family or to the local area in which the family is currently living or has previously lived. Researchers and clinicians should be familiar with possible variants of the words on the *Lista de Vocabulario* [Vocabulary Checklist] and highlight these for parents when appropriate.

Table C.1 lists example substitutes for words provided on the *Lista de Vocabulario* [Vocabulary Checklist]. This is not an exhaustive list. Many other variants may be used depending on dialect, region, or other factors. The dialectal variants listed in Table C.1 were established through various means. First, the parents who completed the forms for the norming study were asked to note any variants. In addition, linguistic informants and research assistants provided examples based on their familiarity with different Spanish dialects. Finally, sociolinguistic sources and dictionaries were consulted in some cases.

ADDITIONAL INSTRUCTIONS FOR *ACCIONES Y PROCESOS (VERBOS)* [ACTIONS AND PROCESSES (VERBS)]

In English, many verb forms are identical to the infinitive form (e.g., *to eat, you eat, they eat*). In Spanish, however, verbs are conjugated into many different forms that differ from the infinitive depending upon person, tense, aspect, and mood (e.g., *comer* [*to eat,* infinitive], *tú comes* [*you eat,* second-person present indicative], *ellos comen* [*they eat,* third-person present indicative], *yo comí* [*I ate,* first-person past indicative]). Many Spanish-speaking parents may not make the connection between the infinitive verb forms presented on the Inventarios and their variants. It is therefore suggested that thc instructions to parents should explain that the verbs are listed in the infinitive form but that in actual talk, verbs can appear in many different forms. Examples of conjugations of many verbs should be presented to parents. Depending on the educational background of the parents, it may be recommended that terms such as *infinitivo* [infinitive] and *conjugaciones* [conjugation] be avoided. The instructions may instead refer to *formas de las palabras* [word forms] or *se dice de maneras diferentes* [the different ways the word is said].

After providing a general overview, it may also be helpful to provide several specific examples. Examples of regular verbs should be chosen from each of the three different endings (*-ar, -er, -ir*), and should sample a variety of forms, including present, past, imperative, and gerund. In addition, several examples of irregular verbs should be given, such as *ir* [to go], *saber* [to know], *hacer* [to do], or *oir* [to hear].

Commonly used examples for each of the verbs listed on the checklist are provided in Table C.2.

Table C.1. Examples of variants for words listed on the *Lista de Vocabulario* [Vocabulary List] of the Inventarios

Inventory I	Inventory II	Section/item	Acceptable variant/substitute
		Sonidos de Cosas y Animales	
•	•	guaguá	uau
		Animales	
	•	bicho	insecto
•	•	borrego	oveja
•	•	búho	lechuza
•	•	mono	chango
•	•	pájaro	pichón
•	•	pescado	pez
•	•	puerco	cerdo, cochino, chancho, marrano
•	•	rana	sapo
	•	víbora	serpiente, culebra
		Vehículos	
	•	autobús	guagua, huahua
•	•	bicicleta	baica
		Alimentos y Bebidas	
	•	chicle	goma
	•	chícharo	pitipúas
•	•	chile	ají, picante
	•	durazno	melocotón
	•	ejotes	vainitas, habichuelas
	•	elote	maíz, choclo
•	•	frijoles	habichuelas
	•	hot cakes	panquéqué
•	•	helado/nieve	mantecado
•	•	naranja	china
•	•	pastel	bizcocho, quéque, torta
•	•	plátano/banana	guineo
•	•	soda/refresco	coca
		Ropa	
•	•	aretes	pendientes
•	•	calcetines/calcetín	media
	•	chancla	sandalia, huarache
•	•	lentes	espejuelos, gafas
•	•	shorts	bermudas
•	•	playera	camiseta
•	•	sombrero	gorra
•	•	vestido	traje
		Partes del Cuerpo	
•	•	oreja(s)	oído(s)
•	•	panza	barriga
		Juguetes	
•	•	pelota	bola, balón
	•	pluma/plumones	bolígrafo
		Utensilios de la Casa	
•	•	basura	zafacón
•	•	botella/mamila	tetera, teta, pacha

(continued)

Table C.1. *(continued)*

Inventory I	Inventory II	Section/item	Acceptable variant/substitute
	•	canasta	cesta
	•	cerillos	fósforos
•	•	cobija	frazada
	•	cubeta	balde
•	•	dinero	chavos, monedas
•	•	fotos	retratos
		Muebles y Cuartos	
•	•	cajón	gaveta
•	•	estufa	cocina, candela
•	•	horno	microondas
•	•	lavabo	fregadero
•	•	recámara	dormitorio
	•	refrigerador	nevera
•	•	regadera	ducha
•	•	televisión	tele
•	•	tina	bañera
		Objetos Fuera de la Casa	
	•	pasto	zacate, hierba
•	•	planta	mata
		Lugares Fuera de la Casa	
	•	cerro	loma
	•	rancho	granja, finca
•	•	tienda/mercado	super
		Personas	
•	•	abuela	nona
•	•	abuelo	nono
•	•	hermana	tata
•	•	hermano	tato
•	•	maestra	seña
		Rutina Diaria, Reglas Sociales, y Juegos	
	•	pon pon tata	cinco lobitos
•	•	tengo manita	que linda manito
•	•	tortillitas	torta de manteca
		Acciones y Procesos	
	•	agarrar	coger
	•	almorzar	lonchar
•	•	dibujar	rayar
	•	platicar	hablar, charlar
		Cualidades y Atributos	
	•	chaparro	bajito
•	•	chico	pequeño
•	•	enojado	enfogonado
	•	morado	violeta, púrpura
•	•	rojo	colorado
	•	tonto	bobo

Table C.2. Examples of variants for verbs listed in *Acciones y Procesos (Verbos)* [Actions and Processes (Verbs)] on the Inventarios

Inventario I	Inventario II	Verb	Sample variant forms
•	•	abrir	abre, ábrelo, abrí
•	•	acabar(se)	se acabó, acábatelo
	•	acompañar	¿me acompañas?
	•	acostar(se)	acuéstate, se acostó
	•	agarrar	agárralo
	•	almorzar	vamos a almorzar, ya almorcé
	•	amarrar(se)	amárrate, me amarré
	•	andar	ándale
•	•	apagar	apágale, se apagó
•	•	apurar(se)	apúrate
	•	arreglar(se)	arréglamelo, ya lo arreglé
	•	asustar(se)	me asusté, se asustó
	•	aventar	aviéntamelo, avienta
•	•	ayudar	ayúdame, ayuda
	•	bajar(se)	bájate, bájame, bajó
•	•	bailar	baila, bailó
	•	barrer	barre, barrió
	•	besar	bésame, besó
•	•	brincar	brinqué, brinco
	•	buscar	busqué, busca
	•	caber	no cabe
•	•	caer(se)	se cayó, cae
	•	callar(se)	cállate
•	•	caminar	camina, no quiero caminar
•	•	cantar	canta, canté
	•	cargar	cárgame, me cargas
•	•	cenar	cené, quiero cenar
•	•	cerrar	ciérrale, cerré, cierro
	•	cocinar	cociné
•	•	comer(se)	me lo como, comí, no quiero comer
	•	comprar	vamos a comprar, me lo compras, cómprame
•	•	correr	córrele, corre
	•	cortar	me corté, corta
•	•	dar	dame, me das
•	•	decir	dime, dile
•	•	desayunar	quiero desayunar
•	•	dibujar	quiero dibujar, dibújame
•	•	doler	me duele, me dolío
•	•	dormir(se)	se durmió, duérmete, no quiero dormir
•	•	empujar	empújame, me empujé
	•	encontrar	lo encontré, no lo encuentro
•	•	enseñar	enséñame, me enseñas
	•	entrar	entra, entré
	•	equivocar(se)	me equivoqué
	•	esconder(se)	me escondí, se escondió
•	•	escribir	escribe, escribió
	•	escuchar	escúchame, no me escuchó
	•	esperar(se)	espérame, espérate

(continued)

Table C.2. *(continued)*

Inventario I	Inventario II	Verb	Sample variant forms
	•	ganar	gané, ganó
	•	gritar	no me grites, grita
	•	gustar	no me gusta, me gustó
	•	hacer	hazme, hizo
•	•	ir(se)	se fue, va
	•	jalar	jala, jaló
	•	jugar	juega, jugó, vamos a jugar
	•	juntar	junta
	•	lastimar(se)	me lastimó
•	•	lavar(se)	se lava, me lavé
•	•	leer	léeme, leí
	•	levantar(se)	me levanté, levántate
•	•	llevar(se)	llévame, llévatelo
•	•	llorar	no llores, lloró
	•	llover	llueve, está lloviendo, llovió
•	•	meter(se)	se metió, mételo
•	•	mirar	mira
•	•	mojar(se)	no te mojes, se mojó
•	•	morder	no muerdas, me mordió
	•	nadar	nada, está nadando
	•	oir	oye, oí
•	•	parar(se)	párate, se paró
	•	patear	pateó, patea
	•	patinar	patina
•	•	pegar(se)	me está pegando, no me pegues
•	•	peinar(se)	péinate, me peinas
	•	pensar	pienso, piensa
	•	perder	se perdió
•	•	pintar	pinta, está pintando
	•	platicar	platícame, platiqué
•	•	poder	no puedo, pude
	•	poner(se)	ponlo, puse
•	•	prender	préndele, lo prendí
	•	quedar(se)	se quedó, quédate
	•	quemar(se)	se quemó, me quemé
•	•	querer	quiero, quieres
	•	quitar(se)	quítatelo
	•	regalar	me lo regaló, regálame
•	•	romper	se rompió, rómpelo
	•	saber	no sé, supo
•	•	sacar	saca, sacó
	•	saltar	salta
	•	salir(se)	se salió
	•	saludar	saluda
•	•	secar(se)	sécate, me sequé
•	•	sentar(se)	se sentó, siéntate
•	•	soplar	sóplale, ya le soplé
•	•	subir(se)	no te subas, me voy a subir
	•	tapar	tápame
•	•	tener	tengo, tiene

Inventario I	II	Verb	Sample variant forms
	•	terminar	ya terminé
•	•	tirar	lo tiré
•	•	tocar	no lo toques
•	•	tomar(se)	ten, tómalo
•	•	trabajar	a trabajar, trabajó
	•	traer	tráetelo
	•	venir(se)	ven, vino
•	•	ver(se)	ve, lo vi

D

SCORING EXAMPLES FOR INVENTARIO I

Appendix D provides snapshots of several sections of Inventario I that have been completed with fictitious data. These example sections are intended to illustrate the procedures used for scoring Inventario I. A more detailed description of scoring procedures and additional information are provided in Chapter 2.

Scoring example: Scoring the *Lista de Vocabulario* (Inventario I) to calculate *Comprensión de Palabras* and *Producción de Palabras*

2. *Animales (de Verdad y de Juguete)* (36)

	comp.	comp. y dice		comp.	comp. y dice		comp.	comp. y dice		comp.	comp. y dice
abeja	●	○	conejo	○	○	lobo	○	●	pingüino	●	○
animal	○	●	elefante	●	○	mariposa	●	○	pollito	●	○
araña	○	○	gallina	○	○	mono	○	○	puerco	○	●
ardilla	○	○	gato	○	●	mosca	○	○	rana	●	○
borrego	○	○	guajolote	○	○	oso	●	○	ratón	○	○
búho	○	○	hipopótamo	●	○	pájaro	○	○	tigre	○	●
burro	●	○	hormiga	○	○	pato	○	○	tortuga	●	○
caballo	●	○	jirafa	○	●	perro	●	●	vaca	○	○
cabra	○	○	león	○	●	pescado	○	●	venado	○	○

Comp: 20 (of 36
Prod: 9 (of 36)

3. *Vehículos (de Verdad y de Juguete)* (9)

	comp.	comp. y dice		comp.	comp. y dice		comp.	comp. y dice
avión	●	●	camión de bomberos	●	○	carro/coche	○	●
barco	○	●	camión/troca	●	○	moto	●	○
bicicleta	○	●	carreola	○	○	tren	●	○

Comp: 8 (of 9)
Prod: 4 (of 9)

4. *Alimentos y Bebidas* (30)

	comp.	comp. y dice		comp.	comp. y dice		comp.	comp. y dice		comp.	comp. y dice
agua	○	●	dulce	●	●	manzana	●	○	queso	●	○
arroz	○	●	frijoles	●	○	naranja	○	○	salchicha	●	○
atole	○	○	galleta	●	○	pan	●	○	soda/refresco	●	○
café	○	○	helado/nieve	●	○	paleta	○	○	sopa	●	○
carne	○	○	huevo	●	○	pastel	●	○	tortilla	●	○
cereal	○	○	jamón	○	○	plátano/banana	●	○	uvas	●	○
comida	○	○	jugo	○	○	pollo	●	○			
chile	○	○	leche	●	○	quesadilla	●	○			

Comp: 20 (of 30
Prod: 3 (of 30)

5. *Ropa* (19)

	comp.	comp. y dice		comp.	comp. y dice		comp.	comp. y dice		comp.	comp. y dice
aretes	○	○	calzón	●	○	pantalón	○	○	sombrero	●	○
babero	○	○	cierre	●	○	pañal	●	○	suéter	○	○
botas	○	○	collar	●	○	pijama	○	○	vestido	●	○
botón	○	○	falda	●	○	playera	●	○	zapato	○	○
calcetines	●	○	lentes	●	○	shorts	○	○			

Comp: 10 (of 19
Prod: 0 (of 19)

Scoring example: Scoring *Gestos y Acciones* (Inventario I) to calculate *Gestos Tempranos*

IIª Parte: Gestos y Acciones

A. Primeros Gestos

Instrucciones: Cuando un niño/a pequeño/a empieza a comunicarse, frecuentemente usa gestos para dar a entender sus necesidades. Por favor, rellene el círculo en la columna correspondiente de los gestos o acciones que su hijo/a haga en este momento.

	todavía no	de vez en cuando	muchas veces
1. Extiende su brazo para mostrarle algo que tiene en la mano.	○	○	●
2. Trata de alcanzar o darle algún juguete u objeto que tiene en la mano.	○	○	●
3. Señala (con la mano y el dedo índice extendidos) algún objeto o situación.	○	●	○
4. Dice "adiós" con la mano cuando alguien se va sin que se le pida que lo haga.	○	○	●
5. Levanta los brazos para que lo levanten.	○	●	○
6. Hace el gesto de "no" con su cabeza.	○	○	●
7. Hace el gesto de "sí" con su cabeza.	●	○	○
8. Hace el gesto de "shhh" (callar) con su dedo enfrente de la boca.	○	○	●
9. Extiende su mano, a veces acompañado de un gemido u otro sonido para pedir algo.	○	○	○
10. Avienta besitos.	○	○	●
11. Aprieta los labios como manera de decir "mmmm" cuando algo está sabroso.	●	○	○
12. Levanta los hombros y/o extiende sus manos hacia los lados como para decir "dónde está" o "se fue".	○	●	○
13. Llama a alguien con la mano haciendo el gesto de "ven".	○	●	●

Yes: 10 (of 13)
No: 3 (of 13)

B. Juegos con Adultos y Rutinas

¿Ha visto a su hijo/a hacer algunas de las siguientes actividades?

	sí	no
1. Juega tortillitas.	○	●
2. Hace ojitos.	●	○
3. Juega acerrín.	●	○
4. Juega pon pon tata.	●	○
5. Juega a esconderse o a corretearse.	●	○
6. Juega a las cosquillitas.	●	○
7. Hace sana sana.	○	○
8. Baila.	●	○

Yes: 6 (of 8)
No: 2 (of 8)

E

SCORING EXAMPLES FOR INVENTARIO II AND SCORING GUIDELINES FOR *M3L-PALABRAS* [M3L-*WORDS]

Appendix E provides snapshots of several sections of Inventario II that have been completed with fictitious data. These example sections are intended to illustrate the procedures used for scoring Inventario II. A more detailed description of scoring procedures and additional information are provided in Chapter 2.

Appendix E also provides detailed instructions on calculating *M3L-Palabras* [M3L-*Words] from the example utterances provided by parents who indicate on Inventario II that their child is combining words.

Scoring example: Scoring the *Lista de Vocabulario* (Inventario II) to calculate *Producción de Palabras*

5. *Ropa* (28)

abrigo	○	calcetín	○	gorra	○	playera	○
aretes	●	calzón	●	guantes	○	ropa	○
babero	○	camisa	○	lentes	○	shorts	○
bolsa	●	cierre	○	medias	○	sombrero	●
botas	○	collar	○	pantalón	●	suéter	○
botón	○	chancla	○	pañal	●	vestido	○
bufanda	●	falda	○	pijama	●	zapato	●

Prod: 9 (of 28)

6. *Partes del Cuerpo* (27)

barba	●	chichi/pecho*	○	mano	●	pelo	○
bigote	●	dedo	○	nalgas*	○	pene*	○
boca	○	dientes	●	nariz	●	piernas	●
brazo	○	garganta/anginas	○	ojos	●	pies	○
cabeza	●	hombro	●	ombligo	●	rodilla	○
cachete	●	labios	○	oreja	○	vagina*	○
cara	○	lengua	○	panza	●		

*o la palabra que use su familia para esto

Prod: 12 (of 27)

7. *Juguetes* (18)

bat	○	hoja/papel	○	osito	○	pluma/plumones	○
burbujas	○	juguete	●	patines	●	tambor	○
colores	○	lápiz	○	pelota	○	triciclo	○
crayolas	●	libro	○	pinturas	○		
globo/bomba	●	muñeca	●	plastilina	○		

Prod: 5 (of 18)

Scoring example: Scoring *Complejidad de Frases* (Inventario II)

C. Complejidad de Frases

A continuación encontrará pares de frases. Por favor señale la que más se parezca a la forma en como hable su hijo/a, en este momento. Si su hijo/a usa frases más largas o complicadas de las que vienen en los ejemplos, por favor marque la segunda frase. El niño/a no tiene que decir exáctamente la misma frase; lo que le pedimos es que marque la frase que se parezca más a la manera en que su hijo/a habla.

No.	Frase	Marca
1.	nene quiere	○
	quiero paleta	●
2.	tuyo esto	●
	este es tuyo	●
3.	Tito malo	●
	soy malo	○
4.	Pepe uvas	●
	quiero uvas	○
5.	agua vamos	●
	vamos al agua	○
6.	a silla	●
	en la silla	○
7.	pollo no	○
	no quiero pollo	●
8.	Paloma llorando	●
	Paloma está llorando	○
9.	mío lápiz	●
	éste es mi lápiz	○
10.	más leche	●
	dame más leche	○
11.	papo mami	●
	el zapato es de mami	○
12.	no aquí	○
	ése no está aquí	●
13.	rompió globo	●
	se rompió el globo	○
14.	leche caliente	●
	la leche está caliente	○
15.	duele panza	●
	me duele la panza	○
16.	guaguá grande	●
	tengo un perro grande	○
17.	calle allá está	○
	allá está la calle	●
18.	puse a mano	●
	lo puse en mi mano	○
19.	acabó agua	●
	se me acabó el agua	○
20.	fue casa	●
	se fue a su casa	○
21.	silla subir	●
	me quiero subir a la silla	○
22.	Marta papá	●
	quiero ir con papá	○
23.	bravo Tello circo	○
	dije bravo en el circo	●
24.	papá calle	●
	papá se fue a trabajar	○
25.	ya puse	○
	ya se lo puse	●
26.	Chalo osito coche	●
	Chalo dejó el osito en el coche	○
27.	lápiz dibujar	●
	dibujo con el lápiz	○
28.	ya pinté	●
	ya acabé de pintar	○
29.	nene rompió bici Danny	●
	el niño rompió la bici de Danny	○
30.	pone no	●
	no lo pongas	○
31.	vamos comer papas carne	●
	vamos a comer papas y carne	○
32.	niño llora cayó	○
	el niño llora porque se cayó	○
33.	mamá nene compra	○
	mamá y nene fueron a comprar	○
34.	abre dame galleta	○
	abre la caja y dame una galleta	○
35.	no toca, quemas	○
	no lo toques porque te quemas	○
36.	quiero libro papá	○
	quiero el libro que compró papá	○
37.	pongo agua flores	○
	pongo agua para que crezcan las flores	○

Number of times more complex phrase is marked: 8 (of 37)

SCORING GUIDELINES FOR *M3L-PALABRAS* [M3L-*Words]

In Part II of Inventario II, *Oraciones y Gramática* [Sentences and Grammar], parents are instructed to write the three longest utterances or sentences they have recently heard their child say. If a parent has indicated that the child is not yet producing word combinations (*Combinación de Palabras* [Combining]) and has not provided example sentences, *M3L-Palabras* [M3L-*Words] cannot be computed directly, but the child is given a default score of 1 (i.e., the child is only producing single-word utterances). If the parent has indicated that the child is producing multiword utterances *de vez en cuando* [sometimes] or *muchas veces* [often] but has not provided sentences, the parent should be contacted to give examples. If that is not possible, then the score should be considered missing and should not be included in any data or evaluation. As noted in Chapter 2, the CDI Scoring Program automatically calculates the *M3L-Palabras* [M3L-*Words] score when the example sentences are entered according to the guidelines in this appendix This is the only part of the Inventarios for which some proficiency in Spanish is needed for scoring.

M3L-Palabras [M3L-*Words] is computed by deriving the mean length in words (rather than morphemes) over the three sample utterances. A *word* is defined as a meaningful string of letters bound by spaces, except for songs, routines, and parent explanations. (See Table E.1 for specific exceptions and examples.) First, count the number of words in each of the utterances provided. Then, sum the individual scores and divide by 3 (or the appropriate number if fewer than three utterances were provided). The resulting number is the child's *M3L-Palabras* [M3L-*Words] score. To obtain a percentile equivalent score, compare the child's *M3L-Palabras* [M3L-*Words] score with those in the percentile table according to the child's age. See Table 5.25 in Chapter 5 to compare the child's score with those of all children in the norming sample. If a gender-specific score is required, use Table 5.26 if the child is a girl or Table 5.27 if the child is a boy. (See the section in Chapter 2 called "Using the Norms" for more information about using the percentile tables and interpreting a child's score.)

SELECTING UTTERANCES TO SCORE

If the parent has written *more than three utterances* on the form, select the three utterances that contain the *greatest* number of words. If fewer than three examples are provided, compute *M3L-Palabras* [M3L-*Words] based on the number of utterances available (one or two).

Check that the parent has written *only what the child says* and not an explanation of what the child does. For example, a parent might write *"solo dice, muy bien papá, mamá, teta, Batman."* In this case, exclude the parent's explanation (*"solo dice"*), and score only the child's utterances (e.g., *"muy bien papá," "muy bien mamá"*).

Table E.1. *M3L-Palabras* [M3L-*Words] scoring examples

Example as written on Inventario II	Word count	Explanation
Quero cobija	2	
Más agua	2	
Mio lápiz	2	
Hola ***Abuela Tita***	2	*Abuela Tita* is a proper noun (1 word).
Pum cayó	2	
*Popa cleo—****refiriéndose al perro del vecino***	2	Parent's explanation is not counted.
Hola ***buenos días***	2	*Buenos días* is a routine (1 word).
Akita *bebé*	2	*Akita* is child version of *aquí está* (1 word).
Dame *pollo*	2	The clitic *me* is not counted separately because *dame* is a routine (1 word).
Buenos días*. ¿Ya* ***te*** *levantas****te****?*	1, 3	Counted as two utterances. *Buenos días* is a routine (1 word); the first (but not the second) *te* is counted separately.
Ay *papá fuchi*	3	The exclamation *ay* is counted as 1 word.
Mira mira *mi pelota*	3	*Mira* is counted only once because it is contiguously repeated.
éste mira éste	3	*Éste* is counted twice because it is noncontiguously repeated.
Mami cantamos ***'estas son las mañanitas'***	3	The name of the song (*estas son las mañanitas*) is counted as 1 word.
Am ti baco	3	These are child words.
Guaguá *pata pito*	3	*Guaguá* is a routine (1 word).
Abue Paulina *me pegó*	1, 3	*Abue* and *Paulina* should be separated by a comma (even though the parent did not write it) to indicate that *Abue* is a vocative and thus is a separate utterance.
Quítate *maña, vete*	3, 2	Counted as two utterances. *Quítate* (clitic) is two words.
Cárgame mami, aquí me pegó Paul	3, 4	This expresses two ideas and should be counted as two separate utterances.
fui a México, fui a casa de abuela y a mi casa de mis primas	3, 12	This expresses two ideas and should be counted as two separate utterances.
Gibo ***(su hermano)*** *está es escuela*	4	Parent's explanation is not counted.
Aquí está *el perro*	4	The parent reported *aquí está* (2 words) rather than the child form (*akita*).
Mami te quiero mucho	4	
Mami quiero una tortilla	4	
Quiero libro compres mami	4	
Adios, dormir mami magos	4	This phrase should not be divided into two utterances, since only one idea is expressed.
Me lo das ***por favor***	4	*Por favor* is a routine (1 word).
Nacho se subió ***ala*** *mesa*	6	*Ala* should be counted as 2 words because the parent has incorrectly written two words (*a la*) as one (*ala*).
Vámonos *en el coche a Querétaro*	6	*Vámonos* is a routine (1 word).
El señor me tomó fotos en misa	7	
Te quiero mucho y a mis hermanas	7	
Toyita mida fuimos a ved a ditor y taba malo	10	The sentence is written the way the child speaks but should still be counted (adult form is *Toyita mira fuimos a ver al doctor y estaba malo*).
Lorena me dio un beso porque era bonito y me peine	11	
Te acuerdas venimos ***al*** *parque con Jude, Fer y Bety*	11	The contraction *al* counts as 2 words.
En el circo bio ***al*** *lobo se quiera comer a los cochinitos.*	13	The contraction *al* counts as 2 words.
Había una vez *una familia de osos que vivián en una casa en medio del bosque*	14	*Había una vez* is a routine (1 word).
Me regañaron ***por que*** *tiré la comida en la silla pero fue un niño yo no*	15	The words *por que* should be counted as *porque* (1 word).

Exclude any utterances that are entirely routines (segments of songs, nursery rhymes, or poems), such as *"Estas son las mañanitas," "tengo manita . . ." "Tortillitas de manteca . . ."* or *"Dale dale dale no pierdas el tino . . ."* ***Note:*** If only part of an utterance that the parent has written is a routine or song, count the routine as one word, and score the remaining words in the utterance as appropriate. For example, if the parent writes *"Mami, en la escuela cantamos estas son las mañanitas,"* count the routine (*"estas son las mañanitas"*) as one word and the remaining words as separate words (total length = six words).

Count any of the following as a *single* utterance:

- Any utterance that consists of more than one independent clause and is connected by a conjunction such as *y* or *o*
- Any utterance with multiple instances of the word *y, y luego,* or *entonces,* such as *"Toyita y yo fuirmos a ver al doctor y estaba enfermo de gripa"*
- Any utterance that contains punctuation marks, if there is no separation of ideas, such as *"no, Omar, no"* or *"mami, más leche"*
- Any utterance that contains two or more subordinated phrases that contrast ideas or express parallel ideas, such as *"me regañaron porque tiré la comida en la silla pero fue un niño yo no"* or *"no quiero comer sopa, quiero pollito y arroz y catsup"*
- Any utterance that contains a tag question, such as *"¿es mío, verdad?"*

Count the following as *separate* utterances:

- Independent clauses that are not connected by a conjunction such as *y* and that express separate ideas but are separated by a comma, colon, or semicolon; for example, if the parent writes *"quítate maña, vete,"* the utterances should be counted as two separate examples (*"quítate maña"* and *"vete"*)
- Utterances that have been written on the same line but that express separate ideas (whether or not the parent has written punctuation marks); for example, *"tío ven mami no puedo"* should be transcribed as two utterances (*"tío ven"* and *"mami no puedo"*)

COUNTING WORDS

Do *not* count words that the parent writes down to *explain* the child's utterance. For example, if the parent writes *"guaguá (dame) pata rapidito,"* do not count *"dame."*

Child words should be counted as words even if they cannot be understood by the scorer, such as *"am ti baco," "guaguá pata pito," "eder titi llorando,"* or *"ota vies gol."*

All *clitics* should be counted as separate words, *except* when in routines, such as *dame, vámonos, ándale,* and so forth. Clitics, in Spanish, are pronominal forms for direct or indirect objects that may accompany verbs. When the verb is conjugated, the clitic antecedes the verb. With nonfinite forms and imperatives, it is attached in the final position. Clitics are marked for their function (e.g., direct/indirect object, middle forms, reflexives) as well as for gender and number, such as with ***me*** *voy, cóme**lo**,* and *voy a guardar**lo**.* Clitics (e.g., *se, le, les, la, lo, las, los, te, me, nos*) may appear within a word (e.g., *ve**te***) or separately (e.g., ***te*** *doy*).

If the parent has separated a word into two words or misspelled a word, *count the word as it should be written.* For example, a parent might write *"a fuera"* instead of *"afuera."* In this case, the correct form, *afuera,* should be used for scoring.

A *frozen phrase or routine* (e.g., *por favor; buenos días; buenas noches; bye-bye; a ver; otra vez; había una vez; al agua patos; uno, dos, tres*) should be counted as a single word, even if it consists of more than one word. It is well known that such phrases function as single lexical units in child language, even though that may not be the case in adult language. Compound words, such as *cepillo de dientes* and *camión de bomberos,* are also considered as single units and should be given a count of one.

- The question form *por qué* should be counted as a single word.
- The word *akita* (child version of the phrase *aquí está*) should be counted as a single word, unless the parent has written the separate words *"aquí está."*
- Proper nouns (e.g., *Pablo Picasso, Abuela Tita*) each should be counted as a single word.

Contiguous repetitions of a word within an utterance (e.g., *"Mira mira mi pelota"*) should be counted only once. If there is a separation between the repetitions (e.g., *"éste mira éste"*), however, each repetition should be counted as a single word.

- Repetitions of conjunctions such as *y, o,* and *entonces* should be counted separately, unless they are contiguous.
- Repetitions of the same word in different utterances should be counted separately. For example, *vamos* would be counted separately in the phrases *"vamos al coche," "vamos al parque,"* and *"vamos a jugar."*
- The contracted forms *al* and *del* should each be counted as separate words, because they are each formed by two separate words that can stand alone.

F

DESCRIPTION OF *COMPLEJIDAD DE FRASES* [COMPLEXITY]

The *Complejidad de Frases* [Complexity] section of Inventario II has 37 pairs of phrases. The first phrase of each pair is a more simple form, whereas the second one is a mature form that may consist of more words or may reflect a change in the order or complexity of the elements and/or the types of word combinations. Complexity may also be increased by adding inflected verbs or by adding function words. Table F.1 illustrates the differences between simple and complex sentences.

Table F.1. Structure of paired items on *Complejidad de Frases* [Complexity] (Inventario II)

Item numbers on *Complejidad de Frases* [Complexity]	Simple structure (first in pair)	Mature structure (second in pair)
1–10	Word juxtaposition (primarily noun–noun)	Verbs and verb inflections
	Noncanonical word order	Canonical word order
11–20	Short phrases	Longer phrases with function words, such as prepositions, clitics (see Appendix E for a discussion of clitics), and articles
21–30	Noun–noun juxtaposition	Verb and verb inflections
	No predicate	Predicates with function words in simple phrases, such as periphrastic verbal phrases, negative imperatives, and prepositional phrases
31–37	Short phrases	Longer phrases with function words
	Short phrases, noun juxtaposition	Combined phrases with connectives, such as *porque, que,* and prepositions

G

CHILD REPORT FORMS/ *INFORMES DEL NIÑO/A*

MacArthur INVENTARIOS

Child Report Form
Primeras Palabras y Gestos (Inventario I)

ID number ________ Date of report ________ Date Inventario completed ________

Child's name ________ (FIRST, MIDDLE, LAST) Child's birth date ________

Parent/guardian ________ (FIRST, LAST) Gender ____ Child's age in months ____

Iª PARTE: PRIMERAS PALABRAS [PART I: EARLY WORDS]

Comprensión Temprana [First Signs of Understanding]

			Percentage of "yes" answers at this child's age (see Table 4.6 in the *User's Guide and Technical Manual)*
Responds when name is called:	☐ yes	☐ no	______
Responds to "no":	☐ yes	☐ no	______
Responds when "papá/mamá" is called:	☐ yes	☐ no	______

Comprensión de las Primeras Frases [Phrases Understood]: Number: ______ (of 28) Percentile: ______

Maneras de Hablar [Starting to Talk]

			Percentage of "yes" answers at this child's age (see Table 4.9 in the *User's Guide and Technical Manual)*
Imita [Imitation]:	☐ yes	☐ no	______
Nombra [Labeling]:	☐ yes	☐ no	______

Lista de Vocabulario [Vocabulary Checklist]

Comprensión de Palabras [Words Understood]:	Number: ______ (of 428)	Percentile: ______
Producción de Palabras [Words Produced]:	Number: ______ (of 428)	Percentile: ______

IIª PARTE: GESTOS Y ACCIONES [PART II: ACTIONS AND GESTURES]

Primeros Gestos [Early Gestures] (A–B)	Number: ______ (of 21)	Percentile: ______
Gestos Tardíos [Later Gestures] (C–E)	Number: ______ (of 43)	Percentile: ______
Total de Gestos [Total Gestures] (A–E)	Number: ______ (of 64)	Percentile: ______

MacArthur INVENTARIOS

Child Report Form
Palabras y Enunciados (Inventario II)

ID number ______________ Date of report ____________ Date Inventario completed ____________

Child's name ________________________________ Child's birth date ________________
FIRST MIDDLE LAST

Parent/guardian ______________________________ Gender ____ Child's age in months ____
FIRST LAST

Iª PARTE: EL USO DE PALABRAS [PART I: WORDS CHILDREN USE]

Lista de Vocabulario [Vocabulary Checklist]

Producción de Palabras [Words Produced]: Number: ______ (of 680) Percentile: ______

Cómo Usa y Comprende el Niño/a el Lenguaje [How Children Use Words]

			Percentage of "yes" answers at this child's age (see Table 4.19 in the *User's Guide and Technical Manual)*
Pasado [Past]:	☐ yes	☐ no	______
Futuro [Future]:	☐ yes	☐ no	______
Objeto Ausente [Absent Object (Production)]:	☐ yes	☐ no	______
Objeto Ausente [Absent Object (Comprehension)]:	☐ yes	☐ no	______
Dueño Ausente [Absent Owner]:	☐ yes	☐ no	______

IIª PARTE: ORACIONES Y GRAMÁTICA [PART II: SENTENCES AND GRAMMAR]

Formas de Verbos [*Verb Forms]

Presente [*Present]: Number of "yes" answers: ______ (of 12)

Pasado [*Past]: Number of "yes" answers: ______ (of 6)

Imperativo [*Imperative:] Number of "yes" answers: ______ (of 6)

Combinación de Palabras [Combining] ☐ yes ☐ no

Percentage of "yes" answers at this child's age (see Table 4.22 in the *User's Guide and Technical Manual):* ______

Ejemplos [Examples]

Length in words of child's three longest utterances: 1. ______ 2. ______ 3. ______

M3L-Palabras [M3L-*Words]: ______ Percentile: ______

Complejidad de Frases [Complexity]

Number of times the more complex sentence is selected: ______ (of 37) Percentile: ______

MacArthur INVENTARIOS

Informe del Niño/a
Primeras Palabras y Gestos (Inventario I)

Número de identificación ____________ Fecha del reporte ___________ Fecha del inventario ____________

Nombre del niño/a ________________________________ Fecha de nacimiento ____________
NOMBRE APELLIDO

Padre/custodio legal ________________________________ Sexo ___ Edad del niño/a en meses ______
NOMBRE APELLIDO

Iª PARTE: PRIMERAS PALABRAS

Comprensión Temprana

			Porcentaje de respuestas afirmativas para su edad (véase la Table 4.6 en el *User's Guide and Technical Manual)*
Responde a su nombre:	☐ sí	☐ no	______
Responde cuando se le dice que "no":	☐ sí	☐ no	______
Voltea cuando llaman a su papá/mamá:	☐ sí	☐ no	______

Comprensión de las Primeras Frases Número: ______ (de 28) Percentil: ______

Maneras de Hablar

			Porcentaje de respuestas afirmativas para su edad (véase la Table 4.9 en el *User's Guide and Technical Manual)*
Imita:	☐ sí	☐ no	______
Nombra:	☐ sí	☐ no	______

Lista de Vocabulario

Comprensión de Palabras:	Número: ______ (de 428)	Percentil: ______
Producción de Palabras:	Número: ______ (de 428)	Percentil: ______

IIª PARTE: GESTOS Y ACCIONES

***Primeros Gestos* (A–B)**	Número: ______ (de 21)	Percentil: ______
***Gestos Tardíos* (C–E)**	Número: ______ (de 43)	Percentil: ______
***Total de Gestos* (A–E)**	Número: ______ (de 64)	Percentil: ______

Informe del Niño/a
Palabras y Enunciados (Inventario II)

Número de identificación ____________ Fecha del reporte __________ Fecha del inventario ____________

Nombre del niño/a ______________________________ Fecha de nacimiento ____________
NOMBRE APELLIDO

Padre/custodio legal ______________________________ Sexo ___ Edad del niño/a en meses ______
NOMBRE APELLIDO

Iª PARTE: EL USO DE PALABRAS

Lista de Vocabulario

Producción de Palabras: Número: ______ (de 680) Percentil: ______

Cómo Usa y Comprende el Niño el Lenguaje

			Porcentaje de respuestas afirmativas para su edad (véase la Table 4.19 en el *User's Guide and Technical Manual)*
Pasado:	☐ sí	☐ no	______
Futuro:	☐ sí	☐ no	______
Objeto Ausente (Producción):	☐ sí	☐ no	______
Objeto Ausente (Comprensión):	☐ sí	☐ no	______
Dueño Ausente:	☐ sí	☐ no	______

IIª PARTE: ORACIONES Y GRAMÁTICA

Formas de Verbos

Presente: Número: ______ (de 12)

Pasado: Número: ______ (de 6)

Imperativo: Número: ______ (de 6)

Combinación de Palabras ☐ sí ☐ no

Porcentaje de respuestas afirmativas para su edad (véase la Table 4.22 en el *User's Guide and Technical Manual):* ______

Ejemplos

Longitud (en palabras) de las tres oraciones más largas: 1. ______ 2. ______ 3. ______

M3L-Palabras: ______ Percentil: ______

Complejidad de Frases

Número de veces que se seleccionó la frase mas compleja: ______ (de 37) Percentil: ______

INDEX

Page numbers followed by *t* and *f* indicate tables and figures, respectively.

www.ingramcontent.com/pod-product-compliance
Lightning Source LLC
Chambersburg PA
CBHW050127190325
23540CB00009B/5
* 9 7 8 1 5 5 7 6 6 1 7 8 *